THE BABY MAKER'S GUIDE
TO GETTING PREGNANT

THE BABY MAKER'S GUIDE TO GETTING PREGNANT

FEATURING THE FIVE STEP FERTILITY SOLUTION

Bonus Information Included:
What Your Doctor Didn't Tell
You about Your Fertility

Stacey "The Baby Maker" Roberts PT, MH and
Women's Complementary Health Expert
and
Developmental Editor Katie Klink, PhD, RN

Positive Image Publishing
6650 W State St
Wauwatosa, WI, 53213
Copyright 2017 by Stacey Roberts and Positive Image Publishing
Published with assistance of CreateSpace
All rights reserved.

ISBN: 0998183709
ISBN 13: 9780998183701

DEDICATION

To my patients
I would like to thank my patients first and foremost for trusting
me to be a part of your journey. I am truly blessed to be a part of
helping you regain trust in your body's natural abilities and to
help you create the life that you have always dreamed of.
To my son, Ryan
You truly are an inspiration for everything I do. I strive
to help others create and expand their families because I
couldn't have imagined not having you in my life.
To Katie Klink
Thank you! Your contribution to this book has not only added additional
perspective but also your developmental editing has helped make this
work shine. Your friendship and help means the world to me.

CONTENTS

FOREWORD BY SOPHOS GEROULIS, MD

THE PREMISE OF *The Baby Maker's Guide to Getting Pregnant* is an important one for those dealing with fertility issues and are trying to improve their health. Our understanding of science has and never will be complete. The human condition innately houses natural curiosity, genuine intrigue for the truth, and separation of fact from myth. The latter may seem like a formidable task, but for those of us who are truth seekers, shuffling through volumes of medical information can be the cognitive equivalent of marathon running.

The Baby Maker's Guide to Getting Pregnant and its Five-Step Fertility Solution may make your life much easier. The principles and guidelines presented here may seem deceptively simple, with a blueprint anyone can follow. The guidelines and advice, however, are likely to have powerful health consequences. Unlike prescription medications, the side effects of following the Five-Step Fertility Solution may be increased energy levels, healthier living, the ability to improve functioning at the cellular and hormonal level, a happier life, and, perhaps the best side effect of all, the gift of life.

As a practicing neurologist and Diplomat of the American Board of Psychiatry and Neurology, I wondered what I would have to say about a book on fertility. As a result, this forced me to reflect on my own career and how we approach patient care in allopathic medicine or what you may have come to know as the traditional medical model practiced in today's day and age. There is no argument that practicing medicine has always been a collaborative approach. Ideally, there is no end-all be-all, hence the reason why many people see more than one specialist as each contributes his or her own body of knowledge to wellness. Consider the information that Stacey has provided here your own additional personal consultant. In order for any discipline to move forward, thinking outside of the box is almost mandatory. I followed these guidelines and strongly believe my own fertility issues were overcome and resulted in a healthy child.

The rules of the game are rapidly changing. As the old adage cites, "absence of proof is not proof of absence." Throughout the history of time, many forward thinkers were called into question by their colleagues. The first physician who proposed hand washing to reduce infections was ridiculed by his peers and is now considered a pioneer in aseptic techniques. Albert Einstein met a similar fate of scorn with his radical ideas about space and time but was later vindicated. And let us not forget that at one time, the belief the world was flat, is now an archaic concept almost laughable to think of the naivete.

A powerful new medical model is emerging as we move forward, referred to as epigenetics, which gives scientific support to how our environment both inside and outside of our bodies affect our health. With this new part of the equation, we cannot leave out the powerful ability of our body to heal itself when provided with the nutrients we evolved to consume. Medications, which are all synthetic pharmaceuticals, can cause relative nutritional deficiencies. Additionally, the constant barrage of environmental toxic exposures and our genetically modified food sources are counterintuitive to our DNA. I am excited about what we are referring to as the concept of epigenetics, and Stacey's book, *The Baby Maker's Guide to Getting Pregnant*, addresses key factors that address epigenetic factors that influence health and subsequently, fertility. The conceptual model of "your genes being your destiny" is being called into question. Your family history may no longer be a death sentence like some of us have been told to believe. In fact, through dietary changes, lifestyle modification, and the right amount of exercise more health issues including infertility are preventable and possibly more curable than you know.

The model of thinking our genes program our bodies without some form of conscious or voluntary direction is becoming a dated concept. Rather they steer us into good or poor health based on the choices we make and the experiences we provide ourselves.

You control your destiny. Let the pages in *The Baby Maker's Guide to Getting Pregnant* that follow be an instrumental source for you.

Sophos Geroulis, MD

EDITOR'S PREFACE BY KATIE KLINK, PHD, RN

I INITIALLY MET Stacey while I was in high school as she worked with our volleyball team. At the time, I was a struggling teenage girl dealing with physical and emotional injuries and looking for some direction as I entered into college. Stacey was not only a mentor, but also the big sister I needed to give me clarity and support as I matured into a young woman. She helped me to realize that the strength and perseverance to make my life a great one was already inside me, and I just needed a little encouragement to get it out!

Once she moved to Australia, we lost touch for a few years but rekindled our friendship recently. Once again, she has become the female support source that I needed, as I again was struggling. (This time with fertility issues). Stacey has always been an honest, trustworthy, and dependable person. Not to mention she is funny and charismatic (at least she thinks she is…Okay, I think so too)!

Having dealt with IVF personally, I realized the lack of resources and support for women and couples traveling on the journey. It was made clear, however, through my relationship with Stacey, that there are great opportunities to endure this emotional rollercoaster. *The Baby Maker's Guide* and the Five-Step Fertility Solution are a significant part of not only surviving this process but also learning how to thrive despite the difficulties. Together Stacey and I share the vision that no matter what life brings, good, bad, or ugly, a person can work through the issues with a strong sense of self, a great support system, and when appropriate, a little bit of humor. That is why I am honored to edit this work and be a small part of helping others who are experiencing fertility treatment. It worked for me, so I know it can work for others too. I not only value Stacey as my friend, but also as a professional who touches the lives of her patients and colleagues with integrity and compassion.

Katie Klink, PhD, RN

INTRODUCTION

EVERYBODY SEEMS TO be talking about fertility issues, but if you listen closely, according to the media, it's not good news. The pressure is on, and time is ticking. Have you waited too long, or do you feel you left it too late? Are your eggs too old or your sperm too few and swimming in circles? Are you tired of all the perceived limitations, the bad news, and the seemingly endless conflicting information available to you?

It's time to get clear on what you can do and focus on the possibilities...

The Baby Maker's Guide to Getting Pregnant was written to provide information you can use to empower yourself to take charge of your fertility and actually do something about it. Yes, you do have more control than you have been led to believe, and there are areas you can explore that can enhance your chance to create a viable pregnancy.

When it is not happening, men and women often feel helpless. Empowering yourself and arming yourself with information that can actually help you are key. It is especially important to know what questions to ask your conventional and alternative medical professionals. You will find all of this and more in the pages of *Baby Maker's Guide to Getting Pregnant.*

The Five-Step Fertility Solution™ and the information provided in this book have been associated with over seven thousand babies born to parents who were told it wasn't likely going to happen for them.

After reading this book, I want you to go back to your team of healthcare professionals confident that you can get more out of each session with them and move closer to where you want to go. After reading *Baby Maker's Guide to Getting Pregnant,* my hope is that you stop feeling helpless and know what steps you can take on your own and with help to conceive. Hopefully, you will stop thinking of yourself as a part of a growing epidemic because according to research from statistics from all around the world, fertility in the age group of women who are having the most babies is not in decline. As you will see, more babies are being born in the more mature age groups than ever before. Fertility rate (i.e., number of children per couple) has declined over the years, and teens and young twenty-somethings are having less babies, but more and more women between the ages of thirty and forty-five are having babies than ever before.

I strive for accuracy when passing along information about fertility and fertility issues to our readers and my patients. A healthy conception is our hope for all who have agonized over a negative pregnancy test or a period yet again, month after month. This book was written to give you the material and information to be empowered and more knowledgeable about your situation and to help you optimize your fertility in the process.

For most medical doctors, if you are over thirty-five, you are "old" when discussing your reproductive outlook. This age seems to be the cut-off age for a pregnancy, which really does not correlate with the findings from statistics cited around the world.

Keep in mind, technically, as long as a woman is not in menopause, she has the potential to create a viable pregnancy. Each individual is of course unique, so refrain from lumping yourself into the "my eggs or sperm are too old" category.

Because there are many perceived roadblocks presented to you, you may feel desperate, fearful, and frustrated, especially when faced with the thought that it may not happen for you.

This book contains an arsenal of information that will arm you with simple steps you can implement to take action toward optimizing your health and fertility.

I wish you all the best in your journey and hope you find this book helpful. If you have any questions or comments, or if there is anything I can help you with, please e-mail me at info@naturalfertility.com.

YOUR FERTILITY FOUNDATION

Confused? Frustrated? Or Just Wanting Reliable Information
About Your Fertility That Actually Works?

Start Here!

CHAPTER 1

FERTILITY ISSUES

THE HONEST TRUTH

IS EVERYTHING IN THE MEDIA AND AT MY DOCTOR'S OFFICE THE TRUTH ABOUT MY FERTILITY?

IT BREAKS MY heart every week. Couples come into my office feeling desperate and beaten down. Many of them say, "You are our last chance, our last hope at having a child." "Time is running out," they say, whether they are twenty-five or forty-five. And occasionally I will have someone grab my hand and ask through sobs of desperation, "Can you please help me?" After finally becoming pregnant with her first child after five years of trying, Emma said, "I would have cut my arm off with a butter knife if you told me that would help me get pregnant." I personally have been working with those dealing with fertility issues since 2000, and the fear and desperation is real and is amped up each year.

Dealing with fertility issues can be brutal. The pain is palpable. You feel lost, yet try to remain hopeful. You become angry, yet try to remain optimistic. It is such a roller coaster! But let's look at why this emotional roller coaster is becoming more and more of a ride into despair than a journey that moves toward the creation of life.

First, it's important to state upfront that fertility is not on the decline. As a matter of fact, it is infertility that is declining. According to an article published in *Fertility and Sterility* entitled "Declining Estimates of Infertility in the United States: 1982-2002," data from the National Fertility Survey and the National Survey of Family Growth found that twelve-month infertility in married women between the ages of fifteen and forty-four declined significantly. In the twenty-year period covered by the study, the rate of twelve-month infertility of these women fell from 8.5 percent to 7.4 percent, not fertility.

Researchers from Westfield State College made similar findings. A group of scientists were researching the "fact" that infertility was increasing. After all, this sentiment was everywhere, especially in the media. The researchers wanted to find the science behind the numbers being touted and began to look for more information so they could elaborate on the increase in infertility with scientific means, but as they researched, they were unable to uncover data that supported these claims.

These findings are not exclusive to the United States. Figures released by the Australian Bureau of Statistics reveal more Australian women over forty are having babies than ever before. A record 12,800 babies were born to women over forty in 2011, which is a significant increase from 2001, when there were 7,100 births to women aged forty plus.

Obstetrician Dr. Michael Gannon, president of the Australian Medical Association in WA, said there was good and bad news in the statistics.

For example, in 1965–82, there was clearly a rapid decline in the number of births per year in those aged between thirty and forty-four, which appeared to correlate with pesticide use, such as DDT (which is not banned) and the oral contraceptive pill; but from 1982 to 1995, they found that in the same age group, women between thirty and forty-four, the number of babies born actually increased.

The researchers' conclusion was that "the media does not always reflect the truth." Are you aware that the media may be affecting your beliefs about your fertility today? Think about it. What have you heard in the media or read in a book or magazine that you have taken as "truth" that is perhaps adding to your stress while trying to conceive? Remember, when you are given statistics for the success rates in IVF, they do not provide definitive information about the experience of any individual woman or couple, and success rates are often based on clinical pregnancies, *not* live births. This means that if there was a positive pregnancy test you, go on the "success" list. But if you miscarry the next day, you are still considered one of their "success" statistics.

Beware! Fertility Stats in the Media (and at the Doctor's Office) Are Wrong!

More recent substantiation of the true statistics not normally discussed includes an article published February 19, 2014, in *Huffpost Women*, "The Age Your Fertility Really Begins to Decline—and Why You Shouldn't Freak Out." In this article, Jean Twenge, the author of *The Impatient Woman's Guide to Getting Pregnant*, is quoted saying that "age-related baby panic is based on largely questionable data." While fertility does decline with age, it is not a decline that is so drastic that women in their late thirties should feel that their fertility window is slamming shut like some statistics suggest. As a matter of fact, Twenge points out that the data we read about and hear about in most doctors' offices is based on statistics from two hundred to three hundred years ago. Yep, you read that right—two hundred to three hundred years ago!

You may be used to seeing graphs like this one in your doctor's office that depict a steep decline in fertility anywhere from the late twenties to early or mid thirties.

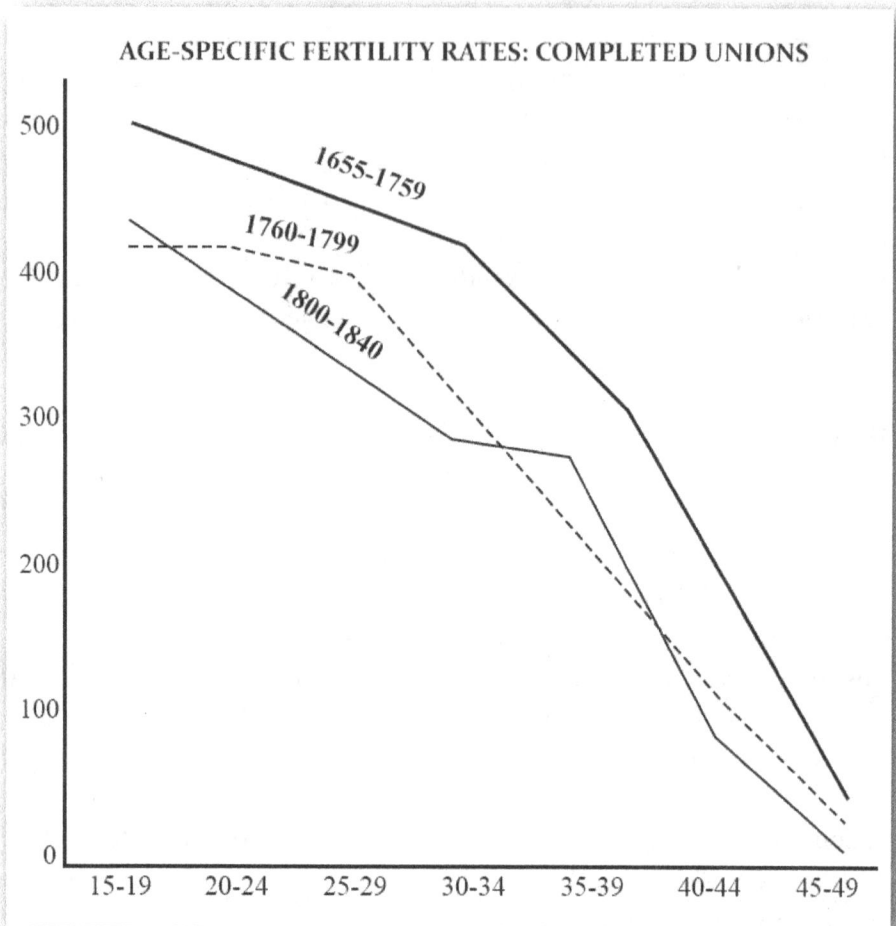

AGE-SPECIFIC FERTILITY RATES: COMPLETED UNIONS

Outdated fertility rates that are still referred to today in many IVF clinics around the world. Robert M. Taylor, Jr. and Ralph J. Crandall, Published by Generations and Change: Genealogical Perspectives in Social History", Chapter 11. Mercer University Press, 1986

However, in the next image you will see the actual birth rates in the United States from the United States Census Bureau survey through 2010

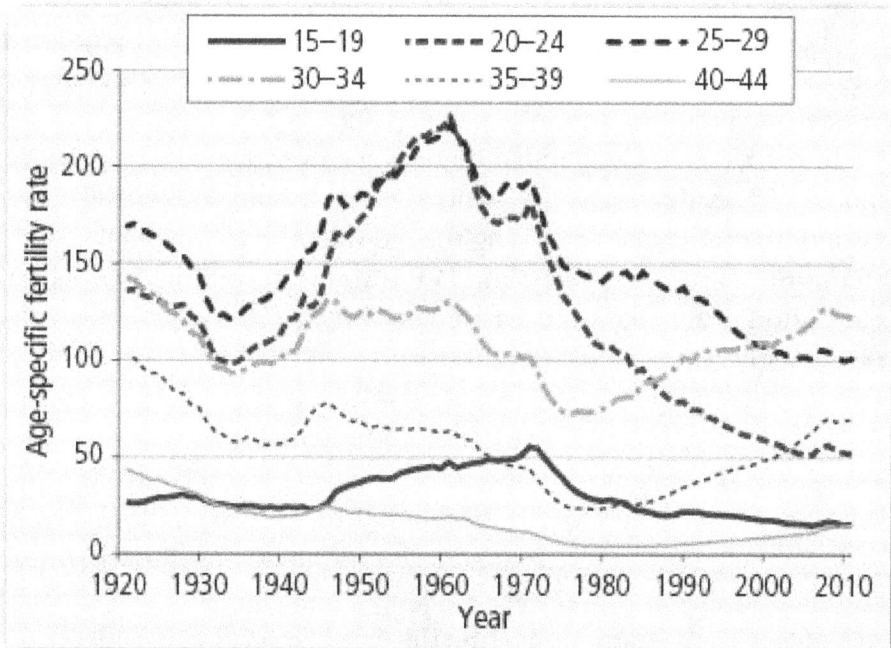

Birth rates per age in the United States

As you can see, the difference between the two graphs is astounding. The first graph from several centuries ago displays statistics from couples who likely did not have running water and electricity. They were also less likely to want more children past the age of thirty or thirty-five. The second graph shows the current trend in birth rates, and as you can see, women are having babies in a much older age range. But which statistics would motivate you to take action? That's right, graph number one. Fear is a powerful motivator, and that is why you have seen graphs like the first one before and will likely see it again and again even though it is significantly out of date.

So what should a man or woman do? Just sit around, do nothing, and keep waiting? Since you are reading this book, clearly you are looking for answers about what you *can* do right now. So the point of me showing you these two graphs is to empower you, not scare you into taking action and to let you know that it may not be too late for you despite how long you have been trying.

Instead, it is recommended that women over the age of thirty-five should seek evaluation by a fertility specialist. But be prepared. Most fertility specialists are still citing the old statistics and will tell you it's all downhill after age thirty, and IVF is your only option. I have over seven thousand babies who have come through my clinic whose parents will give you a very different story.

AGE ALONE DOES NOT DETERMINE YOUR FERTILITY
There are so many factors besides age that impact fertility, and you will find out what they are in this book. In many cases, those factors have a much greater impact on male and female fertility than just chronological age.

Adding to the data supporting the fact that fertility is, indeed, on the rise is a June 17, 2015, *USA Today* article, "Birthrate Among U.S. Women Rises for First Time in Seven Years." While the article initially attributes this increase to an improved economy, the statistics show that a 1 percent increase in fertility and births between 2013 and 2014 cannot be refuted or dismissed. Most interesting among the findings reported is that there has been a 7 percent decline in teen births in each year since 2007—yet overall fertility has still increased. The data was collected from women ranging in age from fifteen to forty-four. With teen births declining at a very significant pace, births to women between the ages of twenty and forty-four have made up for that decline and even surpassed the birth rate by an additional percentage.

THE BILLION-DOLLAR BUSINESS
Let's face it, infertility is a business—a lucrative business at that. In the United States, infertility services are said to be a three billion-dollar business. That is billion with a capital *B*.

And how do many businesses entice you to buy their product? They use fear in their marketing because instilling fear often gets people to take action.

Marketing by instilling fear is a tactic employed by many businesses, and the business of infertility is no exception. Fear-based marketing can be very motivating and results in people purchasing products they never thought they would have to consider and starting procedures much sooner than they thought they would need to.

For example, in 2004, it was very common to have women who were having trouble conceiving wait to complete twelve months of timed intercourse before looking into any issues. Today, if a woman is over thirty-five and trying for six months, she is often told IVF is necessary right away. If a woman is approaching forty or in her early forties, she is often told IVF is her only option and to stop trying naturally and start the procedure immediately. But is this the right step to take?

CHANCES OF GETTING PREGNANT NATURALLY

The numbers to follow represent a woman's chances of getting pregnant after a year of timed intercourse. The statistics are based on age and these can be calculated with the online tool www.countdownto-pregnancy.com Yes the numbers to decline with age but if a woman between 35 and 44 years of age has a 71 percent chance of creating a viable pregnancy with timed intercourse for one to two years, why would doctors be encouraging those couples to pay for an expensive procedure when there is a good chance she will become pregnant in six more months? I am not against IVF, and I refer patients to IVF. But starting a procedure without preparation or when the odds are still in your favor seems a bit too quick based on the stats.

Chance of pregnancy after one year of timed intercourse:
Twenty-five to thirty years old: 96%
Thirty to thirty-five years old: 85%
Thirty-five to thirty-nine years old: 71%

Chance of pregnancy after two years of timed intercourse:
Forty to forty-four years old: 71%
Forty-five to forty-nine: 22%

CHANCES OF GETTING PREGNANT WITH IVF

IVFpredict, developed by Professors Scott Nelson and Debbie Lawlor and available at IVFpredict.com, is a mathematical formula that predicts a couple's chance of having a live birth with IVF. The model used data obtained from more than 144,000 IVF cycles, which shows the chances of a live birth after trying naturally for a year in couples who have no known causes for their fertility issues.

- For a twenty-five-year-old, first IVF attempt 32.4 percent *live births*
- For a thirty-year-old, first attempt: 32.4 percent; second attempt (if first attempt failed): 22.8 percent; second attempt (if first attempt resulted in a birth): 29 percent
- For thirty-five- to thirty-seven-year-olds, first attempt: 26.5 percent; second attempt: 18.2 percent
- For thirty-eight- to thirty-nine–year-olds, first attempt: 19 percent; second attempt: 12.7 percent
- For forty- to forty-two–year-olds, first attempt: 11.4 percent; second attempt: 7.4 percent
- For forty-three- to forty-four-year-olds, first attempt: 4.2 percent; second attempt: 2.6 percent
- For forty-five- to fifty-year-olds, first attempt: 1.7 percent; second attempt: 1 percent

Given those odds, why are doctors strongly recommending women who are older than thirty five go to IVF after six months when she only has a 26 percent chance of a live birth when if she tried for six more months her chance of pregnancy is 71%? Even considering this number would drop off somewhat when calculating live births, her chances would still not drop to 26 percent or less. The following six months could be well spent by couple getting healthier and increasing their chances of conceiving naturally before going to IVF.

Note: At my clinic, we are not against IVF and do refer patients to IVF specialists. We also work directly with IVF clinics to support programs to optimize their patients' health, but we believe patients should make the decision to pursue these avenues (and really any avenue) to optimize their fertility based on what they truly believe makes sense to them—not based on fear-based marketing in the media or at the doctor's office, or because they are so beaten down and disempowered they don't know what else to do. I do not suggest if you are forty that you sit around for two or three years waiting to conceive if you have someone you want to start or expand your family with but to start IVF immediate simply because of your age really doesn't make sense. Later you will see how you can prepare your body for a pregnancy naturally or with IVF.

Sally remembers, "The first time I went to an IVF clinic at thirty-eight for an evaluation, they told me to book in for a procedure my next cycle because time was of the essence. I went into the procedure totally unprepared and foolishly thinking that it would work the first time. It didn't, and I was devastated. After taking six months off to get my head back in the right place, not to mention my body, I responded better to IVF the next stimulated cycle and became pregnant on the frozen embryo cycle a few months later. I felt so much better going into that cycle, I think because I took the time to get myself right."

Supporting couples who want to become pregnant naturally or through IVF is a very important part of the process. When a decision is made out of fear, the desired result rarely ever happens. Getting your body in a healthy, balanced state will help you be able to make your decisions and find clarity among the chaos. If you feel pressured in any way to make a decision, whether it is from a doctor regarding a procedure or a naturopath recommending hundreds of dollars' worth of supplements, unless it makes total sense to you, you don't have to make your decision at that moment. Instead, go away and think about what truly makes sense to you both as a couple.

IMPORTANT QUESTIONS TO ASK

Ask questions about success rates. Are they based on babies born or clinical pregnancies? You will find that the success rates they give you are usually based on pregnancies (which may or may not end up in miscarriage), not live births of healthy babies.

How old are the statistics they are quoting you? If the success rates are very high (higher than what we referenced from ivfpredict. com previously), ask if they are selective about the patients they accept for IVF at their clinic. What is their selection criterion? Do they not include some patients in their analysis of success rates or do they turn away patients if they don't meet certain criteria?

If you are seeing a naturopathy or Chinese medicine practitioner and feel pressured to purchase several hundreds of dollars' worth of supplements, ask specifically what these supplements are for. Are they given to everyone trying to conceive, or are they recommended based on what each person needs on an individual basis? Ask if the herbal formulas are prepared for each individual and their current and past history or if the same standard formulations are given to all patients presenting with fertility issues.

How the practitioner answers these questions should give you essential insight which can help you decide what your next steps should be. If they are open and straightforward with their answers and their answers make sense to you based on statistics, not opinion, and you feel comfortable with them, you are likely in the right place. If they avoid answering your questions or seem bothered by you asking or seem to rush you through an answer you don't understand, you may want to reconsider whether they are the right practitioner for you.

The main issue really is that you feel comfortable that your practitioner is communicating well with you, striving to support you, and assessing any progress with each session you have with them while creating the next step in the plan with you.

Note: Naturopaths and Chinese medicine practitioners may not be able to give you success rates because not all of their patients are going through IVF, and when trying naturally, there is no procedure one day (such as IVF) and an outcome two weeks later to measure. Beware of anyone who says they have a *very* high success rate. As you have seen, even trying naturally, in the general population, for a year will on average be 70 percent live baby rate. Any natural practitioner touting higher numbers than that should be cautiously considered or avoided all together.

CHANGES TO THE FACE OF FERTILITY
There have been many changes in the ages that women give birth over the years as well as the number of births per woman over the last thirty to forty years. However, most of the "your fertility falls off after thirty-five" fertility statistics, as discussed, are based on data obtained centuries ago—data that has been disproven in many aspects today.

Too often, women rely on that data for information about conceiving a child, believing that after the age of thirty, they are considered geriatric when it comes to their fertility.

The facts contradict this belief, and in the United States, statistics show that a very interesting trend has come to light.

A January 2016 article by the United States Centers for Disease Control and Prevention provides us with an update that verifies an increase in the age of mothers in the United States between the years 2000 and 2014. The following data was taken from CDC's "Mean Age of Mothers Is on the Rise: United States, 2000–2014" and provides us with current statistics on fertility according to the age of the mother. Of specific importance are the following findings:

- The average age of mothers in the United States has increased from 2000 to 2014 for all birth orders; the age of first births has increased from 24.9 years to 26.3 years.
- The largest increases in age for births occurred from 2009 to 2014.
- The age increase applied to all states, as well as the District of Columbia, which had a 3.4 year increase in maternal age.
- From 2000 to 2014, first births to women aged thirty to thirty-four rose twenty-eight percent (from 16.5 percent to 21.1 percent), and first births to women thirty-five and over increased 23 percent (from 7.4 percent to 9.1 percent).

The following chart shows the average age of first births by mothers in different age ranges. You can seen a clear increase in those births by all mothers aged twenty-five and older.

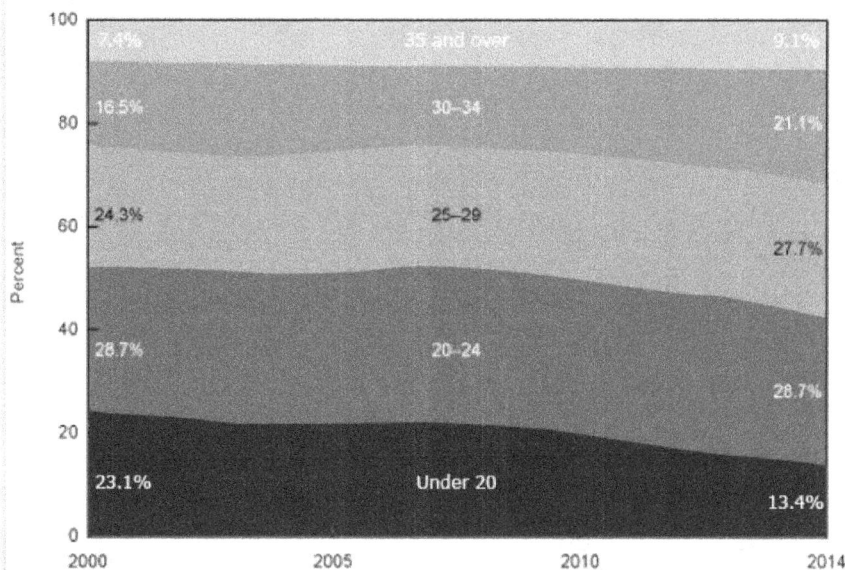

Percentage of first births, by age of mother: United States, 2000–14
SOURCE: CDC/NCHS, National Vital Statistics System

Each individual is unique, and a person's particular situation will result in varied experiences among persons of the same chronological age. While the information here might be directed at certain ages, please understand that all individuals will not fall into the general statistics as there are too many variables to possibly encompass every dynamic. At naturalfertility.com, we consider each person to be an individual. We believe it is not the age but the quality of the eggs, endometrial lining, and the quantity and quality of the sperm that matter most.

CHAPTER 2

ASSESSING FEMALE AND MALE FERTILITY

IF YOU MISSED the section in the last chapter about the fact that the statistics used today are outdated and inaccurate, please go back and read it through. That misleading information is the cause of so much misplaced anxiety and worry, so it is important to understand.

Regarding how female fertility is assessed, we still have a long way to go to develop accurate methods of determining female fertility potential.

Despite what you read, there is no one test that determines how many eggs a woman has left or how healthy they are. If a couple has been trying over twelve months and nothing is happening, even if tests are all normal or they have a specific diagnosis, further assessments than simply the typical blood tests are necessary in order to fully evaluate what may be contributing to a woman's fertility issues. Simply saying "your eggs are too old" or "you are running out of eggs" just doesn't cut it anymore. Couples today want real answers and an effective strategy to help them on their journey to become parents.

As already discussed, as a female ages, she can take somewhat longer to become pregnant. However, in a 2006 article in the medical journal *Reproduction*, the authors stated chronological age is a poor indicator of reproductive aging, and in the last decade, new information has been released that women's eggs are not just gradually getting older and unhealthier for women aged thirty, forty, or fifty years.

Despite this, most of the focus is still on the age of the female, although many studies are now also reporting the age of the male is important. What we see most often, though, especially in IVF circles, is that if the procedure doesn't work, then at least 90 percent of the time, the explanation the couple or female is given is that there is something wrong with the woman's eggs, especially if she is over thirty-five years old even if there is *no* objective evidence (besides the year in her date of birth). The sperm is rarely ever considered to be an issue if a fertilization occurs, even when there are overt, significant issues with the sperm already identified. Always keep in mind the sperm contributes more to a developing embryo than just fertilization. Thankfully, as you will see in the next chapter, research is supporting this as well.

The reality is that the sperm and the egg are both involved in the development of an embryo and whether or not the embryo implants. The sperm's job goes well beyond fertilization. It must be healthy enough to contribute to a viable embryo continuing to develop.

IT'S NOT ALWAYS A FEMALE THING

The medical focus continues to shine mostly on the female's eggs, especially when IVF or other procedures/medications haven't worked. When asked why a couple isn't getting pregnant with IVF or naturally, many fertility doctors will usually say the woman's eggs are too old, although there is no definitive testing to support the truth of this diagnosis. The tests that are relied upon to assess a female fertility potential such as Anti-Mullerian Hormone (AMH) or Follicles Stimulating Hormone (FSH) are often found to be inaccurate and unreliable.

Unfortunately, whether male factor infertility is diagnosed or not, many women will accept the outdated and often incorrect reasoning that her eggs are simply too old or are poor quality without proof. An embryo's development and whether it implants or not relies both on the female *and* the male. When we don't shine the light brightly on this fact, thousands of women live with guilt, anger, sadness, and shame for a long time to come. Many women secretly blame themselves. Many have told me they feel ashamed that they aren't living up to their own expectations or the expectations of their family. They blame themselves for waiting too long to become pregnant, when ironically, for so many years, they did everything possible *not* to become pregnant.

Some physicians tell women that because IVF isn't working, they have a better chance with a donor egg or embryo. At this point, it's important to consider the possibility of a donor, but while you're considering and researching utilizing a donor, which is a completely valid option for many and necessary for some, also ask yourself if you both have done everything to prepare yourselves and optimize your fertility before you attempted the IVF procedure. If not, ask yourself, "What else can *we* do to optimize our chances of using our own eggs or own sperm?" Thankfully, the information you'll find in these pages will help you improve your health and fertility, and if you decided to go with a known donor, our Five-Step Fertility Solution can apply to the donor as well.

Dr. John Rapisarda of Fertility Centers of Illinois in the United States also suggests that a person considering an IVF clinic or the use of a donor should ask about the donor success rates. He calls it the great equalizer among IVF clinics. I would also ask the physician what the live-birth rate for donor embryos is for the year, not just their best week.

⌒

Dr. John Rapisarda explains that the physicians and clinics have different criteria that limit entry into their IVF programs and that the more restrictive criteria leads to higher pregnancy rates because only individuals with the best prognosis are eligible for treatment. "This may then limit access to services for some couples who are less likely to get pregnant, making it difficult to directly compare statistics between programs. At the end of the day, it is important to remember that infertility is a billion-dollar business, and it wouldn't be unheard of in the vastly competitive business of reproductive medicine that some clinics want to beef up their success rates to attract more patients. Be aware and always inquire at another clinic if you are uncomfortable with the advice you are getting."

I believe most doctors who recommend utilizing a donor or canceling a cycle if there was a low response do this because they are concerned for the patient's well being and want to give them the best chance to conceive. However, these decisions are based on their beliefs about a female's age and her egg supply, not about new research that applies to both. As you will see in the next chapter, this belief is based on an old theory that has been challenged in recent studies.

Dr. Jonathon Tilly discovered the possibility that women are not storing their eggs up in their ovaries for years, but instead he and his research team discovered the mechanism by which females create their eggs each month. See more on this in chapter 2.

In my opinion, most times, whether it's been recommended to do another cycle of IVF or a donor cycle, not enough has been done to know why a viable pregnancy isn't occurring. Just like in many parts of medicine today, the reason why something is occurring is not addressed or even fully investigated. Treatment with expensive drugs and surgery often prevail over digging deeper to see how you can address the underlying causes that are affecting your fertility.

Consider Jane: At forty-four years old and after several IVF cycles over the years, she decided to take a break. She took an unprecedented twelve-months to prepare for her last IVF cycle at the age of forty-five. Though you will read in more detail what she did in those twelve months throughout this book, I can tell you now that she conceived and created a baby girl with her own eggs after being told it could never happen. Investigating some oftentimes overlooked areas and addressing those issues is the key to creating a viable pregnancy naturally or with IVF.

MALE AGE AND FERTILITY

In the media in the last few years, there has been a very gradual shift toward considering problems with male age and fertility as well as the effect that a mature male who creates a pregnancy will have on their future child's mental and physical development. After all, it was only in 2005 that paternal age was associated with Down's syndrome; whereas, prior to 2005 and still unfortunately today by those less informed, Down's syndrome was only *assumed* to be associated with maternal age and/or maternal genetic component.

Like their female counterparts, when the Five-Step Fertility Solution™ has been applied to male fertility, in many cases, we have seen an increase in sperm count and improved quality. For many, this progress was followed by a viable conception because, ultimately, a viable conception results from optimal sperm health, optimal egg health, and optimal development and maintenance of the endometrial lining in the uterus.

When asked how age affects male fertility, Dr. Harry Fisch, a professor of clinical urology at Columbia University Medical Center's New York-Presbyterian Hospital and author of *The Male Biological Clock*, stated that testosterone declines as men age and sperm from older men are more likely to cause genetic abnormalities than sperm from younger men. According to Dr. Fisch, after age thirty, testosterone production drops by 1 percent each year, which by itself is not of great significance. However, the biggest problem isn't sperm count—it is a drop in semen volume and the quality, that is, changes in the movement (motility) and shape (morphology) of the sperm. These are all factors that can and do impact fertility.

"Fertility and the Aging Male," a 2011 article published in the *US National Library of Medicine, National Institutes of Health,* supports these claims with findings from the Avon Longitudinal Study of Pregnancy and Childhood. Studying 8,559 pregnancies, this study found that conception within twelve months was 30 percent less likely for men over the age of forty as it was for men under the age of thirty.

A study published in the journal *Fertility and Sterility* revealed that researchers found it takes up to five times longer for a man over forty-five to create a pregnancy with a female than it would if he was under twenty-five. Although the impact of age on a woman's fertility has been under the microscope for years, this was the first time such a strong correlation was found between age and male fertility relating to the time it takes to conceive a child.

"It's always been said that men make sperm every day, and women are born with all the eggs they're going to have, so the effect of male age on fertility hasn't been perceived as a major issue until now," says researcher Stephen Killick, MD, professor of reproductive medicine at the University of Hull, UK. In many cases, "there was just as strong an association with male age and infertility, and in some cases, statistically, it was even stronger than the woman's age."

Killick explains that in a man under twenty, regardless of female age, a pregnancy is likely to occur in 4.5 months; but with a man over fifty, that timeframe increases to twenty-six months. Compared to men who were under twenty-five, men over forty-five were nearly five times as likely to have a time to pregnancy of more than one year and more than twelve times as likely to have a time to pregnancy of more than two years.

Some experts say that age takes its toll on male fertility beginning at age thirty, with a sharper decline after age thirty-five. Thinking that male fertility is preserved because sexual function continues is the wrong assumption. More often scientific research is revealing that lifestyle including what we put in our bodies and the environment around us, not simply age, is impacting the fertility of both sexes.

BASIC SEMEN ANALYSIS *Not* ENOUGH

It is also assumed that a basic semen analysis gives all the necessary information about a male's fertility, but it has been shown that this is not the case. Thankfully there is now proof that a male's fertility is a major factor in the couple's ability to conceive. It's also a fact that typical sperm analysis doesn't address the many factors that impact male fertility, and, therefore, medical professionals don't have sufficient information to determine the proper treatment or therapies. While women are typically subjected to more invasive therapies and treatments, even though they may be fertile, male testing may not go beyond a basic semen analysis, which is very limited in the information it provides, when they are deemed fertile.

This semen analysis can serve a purpose in diagnosing men who have an obvious issue such as very low sperm count, but it fails to fully assess the health of the sperm. The health of the sperm is not represented completely simply by how the sperm swims. The DNA of the sperm, which is often overlooked, is crucial for the sperm to be able to contribute to the development of a healthy embryo after fertilization. Even if the sperm count is off the charts, the quality of the sperm, including motility and whether the DNA is significantly damaged, will determine whether an embryo is likely to go on developing into a healthy baby or whether chances increase for a miscarriage. The same of course is true for the egg.

To rule out the male's contribution to fertility simply because of a normal basic semen analysis is a huge mistake that we see happening every day.

This, much like many female fertility issues, can be addressed with our Five-Step Fertility Solution. More about male fertility will be discussed in chapter 4.

CHAPTER 3

FEMALE-FERTILITY BASICS

THE FOLLOWING SECTION goes over what most people slept through in biology class during high school—the basics of the reproductive system. So grab a little green tea to keep you awake and alert and dive right in.

From this section, I hope you gain an understanding of the intricacies of fertility for both men and women while developing an appreciation for how intelligent our bodies are. When dealing with fertility issues, there are times when you can lose faith and trust you once had in your body when you didn't give a second thought to whether you would be able to conceive.

When you take a moment to learn about the reproductive system, you gain an appreciation for how amazing it really is to create a viable pregnancy. In time you will see there are five crucial steps you can take to help this process along tremendously.

Here we go, back to biology class and Reproduction 101.

THE FEMALE MENSTRUAL CYCLE

In the clinic, whenever I explain what happens during the female menstrual cycle, I am always surprised at how interested both the male and the female are in this topic. When I show them my graphs and pictures, I see a lot of leaning in and nodding and sometimes surprised looks. A few times the guys give me the "too much information" look, but for the most part, both of them are thirsty for knowledge and just want to understand what is going on.

Couples can experience fertility issues for years, but no one ever explains to them the basic components of how it all works.

Gaining an understanding of these basics helps a couple to become empowered and involved in their program. It helps them understand what we are trying to focus on and why, as well as see how the actions in their life can make a difference to their fertility.

FEMALE HORMONE BALANCE: WHAT YOU ABSOLUTELY NEED TO KNOW

The female menstrual cycle consists of two parts. These parts are divided by ovulation, that is, the release of an egg. The first half of the menstrual cycle, up to ovulation, is called the follicular or proliferative, phase. The dominant fluctuating hormones in this phase are FSH, Estrogen (Estradiol), and LH. This is the stage of the menstrual cycle when the follicle and eggs are maturing.

THE FOLLICULAR PHASE

The Female Menstrual Cycle—The Follicular Phase

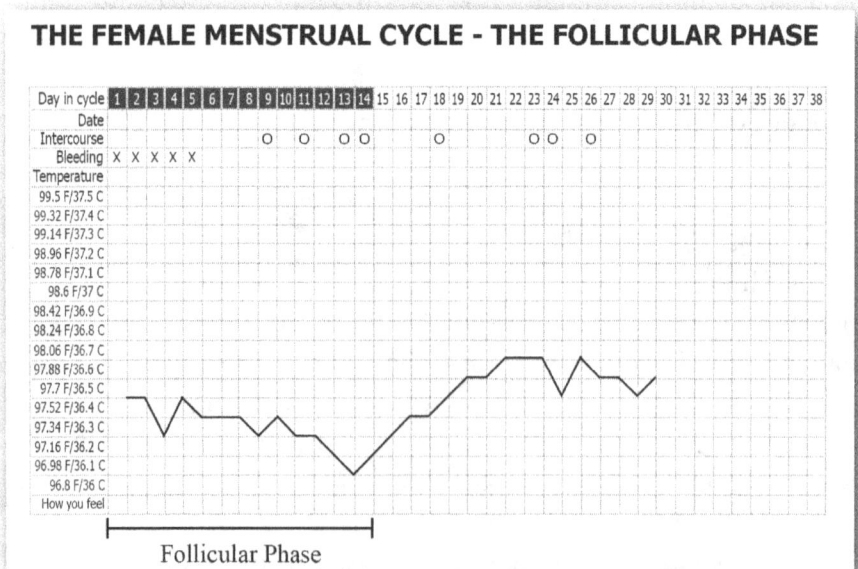

THE FEMALE MENSTRUAL CYCLE - THE FOLLICULAR PHASE

Day in cycle	1	2	3	4	5	6	7	8	9	10	11	12	13	14	15	16	17	18	19	20	21	22	23	24	25	26	27	28	29	30	31	32	33	34	35	36	37	38
Date																																						
Intercourse						O		O		O	O				O							O	O		O													
Bleeding	X	X	X	X																																		
Temperature																																						

Temperature scale (°F/°C):
99.5 F/37.5 C
99.32 F/37.4 C
99.14 F/37.3 C
98.96 F/37.2 C
98.78 F/37.1 C
98.6 F/37 C
98.42 F/36.9 C
98.24 F/36.8 C
98.06 F/36.7 C
97.88 F/36.6 C
97.7 F/36.5 C
97.52 F/36.4 C
97.34 F/36.3 C
97.16 F/36.2 C
96.98 F/36.1 C
96.8 F/36 C

How you feel

Follicular Phase

The follicular phase

FOLLICULAR PHASE AND EGG HEALTH

The first half the menstrual cycle, that is, the follicular phase, begins with a cascade of hormones starting in the brain.

When there is no pregnancy, a hormone called gonadotropin releasing hormone (GnRH) is secreted from the nerve cells of an organ in the brain called the hypothalamus. GnRH travels to an organ in the brain called the pituitary to encourage release of a hormone called FSH (follicle stimulating hormone) to communicate directly with the ovaries.

FSH stimulates the growth of the follicles. LH, or luteinizing hormone, is another hormone that is significant to those wanting to time intercourse because as you will see, it is related to ovulation.

Note: One little known fact is that the follicle takes some time to develop. Some research has shown that the follicle may actually start to develop to eight cycles before it comes up onto the ovary (Stanford University). Remember, eventually the egg is growing up inside the follicle, and just like the house you grew up in had a lot to do with your health, so, too, does the health of the follicle and its contents influence the health of the egg. If you rush into procedures without taking advantage of this development process, you may be creating less healthy eggs and embryos as a result. In other words, this is another reason to consider preparing your body for at least six to eight months prior to trying to conceive.

The last three months of the follicle's development is based on the balance of reproductive hormones and nutritional status.

But now, back to the development of the follicles...

A number of very immature follicles called primordial follicles (with early stage eggs in them) start to develop in the follicular phase and coincide with fluctuations of both FSH and LH from the brain.

Their growth in the later stages is influenced by estrogen and its fluctuations in the first half of the cycle.

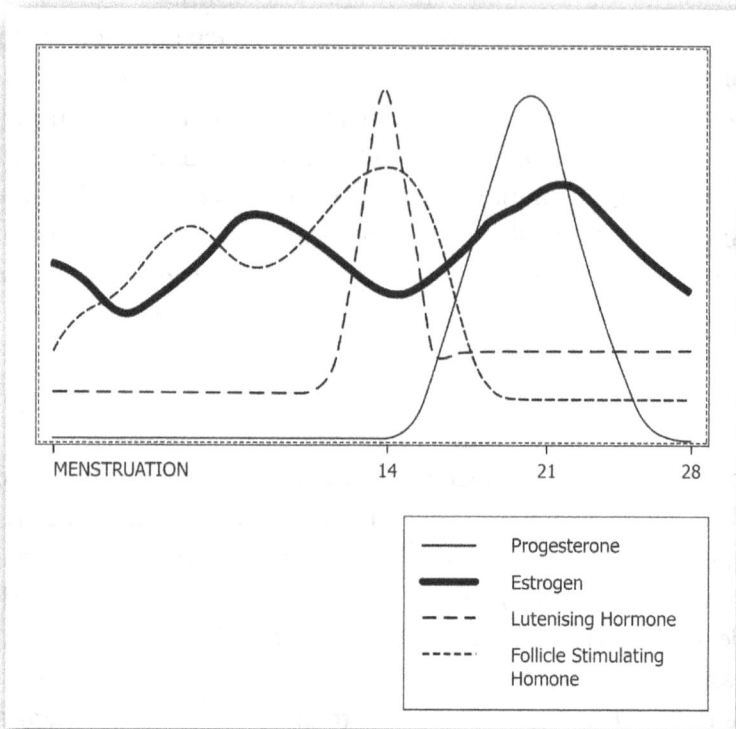

	Progesterone
	Estrogen
	Lutenising Hormone
	Follicle Stimulating Homone

Female hormone balance

During the first few days of the menstrual cycle, FSH is believed
to signal to ovaries to continue the growth of the young follicles (via
estrogen production) to begin developing into mature follicles and
eggs. This can be seen in the next diagram.

One or two dominant follicles develop, and the rest of the follicles
that had originally appeared on that ovary for that particular cycle
get reabsorbed back into the ovary through a process called atresia
(illustrated in the next picture) while the dominant follicle(s) continue to develop. It is as if the dominant follicles send a message to
the other less-developed follicles, saying, "Look, sisters, we've got it

covered this cycle; see ya later!" and the less-developed follicles are reabsorbed back into the ovary. During this time, estrogen begins the development and thickening of the endometrium (lining of the uterus), and further development of the egg and follicle continues.

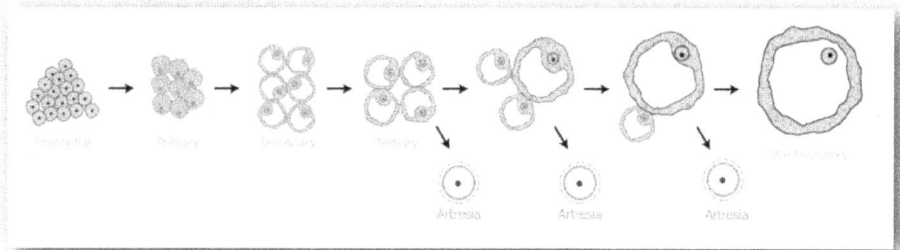

Atresia

Estrogen peaks right before ovulation, which sends a signal to the brain to increase the release of luteinizing hormone (LH surge). This LH hormone surge (also influenced by GnRH) happens, and the egg is released from the follicle.

The dominant follicle in the ovary generally releases an egg around the thirteenth or fourteenth day of a twenty-seven- or twenty-eight-day cycle.

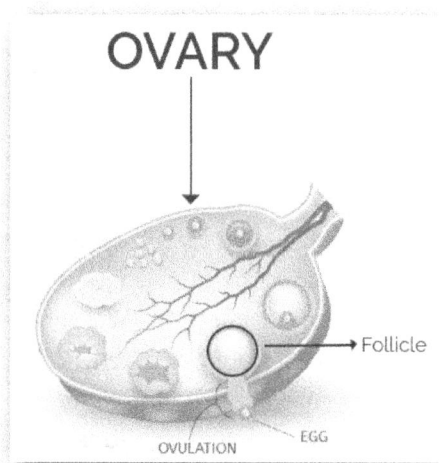

Ovary, follicle, and ovulation

But not everyone's cycle is twenty-seven or twenty-eight days, so the day of ovulation may vary. Some women have very short follicular phases (less than nine days), which could indicate the egg is too immature to be fertilized, and some women have longer follicular phases. A longer follicular phase, if consistent, seems to be less of an issue if the female is following the Five-Step Fertility Solution. However, a longer follicular phase can be more of an issue with conceiving if a woman presents irregular cycles. The irregular cycles make it difficult to know when ovulation is going to happen, and therefore timing intercourse for conception is challenging.

When a woman is diagnosed with polycystic ovaries or recurrent miscarriage, optimizing the length of the long follicular phase (if it is more than twenty days) has proven effective in creating a viable pregnancy in the clinic. Again, this may be due to being able to accurately time intercourse than being related to egg health; nevertheless, optimizing the follicular phase to ten to twenty days in length has correlated with increased viable pregnancies for many women in the clinic.

Have you been told you aren't ovulating even though you are having a period?

The varying length of the follicular phase for women can also create much confusion about whether a woman is ovulating or not.

Sometimes doctors will test to confirm ovulation automatically on day twenty one of the woman's cycle. However, depending on her total cycle length day twenty one may not be the correct day to test. If the doctor doesn't ask about the total length of the cycle, they may assume it is a twenty eight day cycle. If this was the case, most women with twenty eight day cycles would ovulate on day fourteen. Then seven days later is day twenty-one when progesterone should be at its highest level. So for this woman day twenty-one would be a good time to test. But if a woman has a longer or shorter cycle than twenty eight days, testing ovulation on day twenty one may give an inaccurate reading of whether she ovulated or not. You will learn more about this in the next chapter, Determining Ovulation.

THE LUTEAL PHASE AND IMPLANTATION

THE FEMALE MENSTRUAL CYCLE—THE LUTEAL PHASE

The second half of the cycle, called the luteal or secretory phase, occurs after ovulation. At this time the hormone progesterone increases significantly. Progesterone is secreted by the follicle that just released the egg. This structure, which is now called the corpus luteum (scientists probably changed the name just to confuse us), remains present on the ovary and releases progesterone. The increase in progesterone coincides with a rise in temperature after ovulation. See next diagram.

THE FEMALE MENSTRUAL CYCLE - THE LUTEAL PHASE

Luteal Phase

The luteal phase

As you may already know, progesterone enhances the development of the endometrium, that is, the lining of the uterus. If there is no pregnancy, the corpus luteum stops secreting progesterone, and progesterone levels subsequently drop in the last part of the cycle since a conception did not occur. This initiates the coming away of the uterine lining, resulting in the menstrual flow or "period."

If sperm are present and able to get to the egg within twenty-four to forty-eight hours after the egg is released, fertilization could take place. The sperm fertilizes the egg in the fallopian tube. The fertilized egg turns into an embryo, which makes its way into the uterus a few days later and finds a place in the endometrial lining to implant.

If the embryo continues to develop, the implantation of the embryo into the endometrial lining continues. The leftover follicle (remember, it's called the corpus luteum) will continue to make progesterone to maintain the lining and support the pregnancy. The corpus luteum continues to make progesterone in pregnancy until the placenta takes over completely in the second trimester. Up to the first eight to ten weeks of pregnancy, the embryo is receiving its nutrients primarily from the endometrial lining.

Blood flow usually does not exchange from mother and the developing embryo, now called a fetus, until approximately eight and a half to ten weeks. Early pregnancy losses are usually due to a chromosomal abnormality caused by the egg or the sperm, or both. Another reason for early miscarriage is low progesterone. If progesterone does not continue to enhance the endometrial lining, the embryo is at risk of miscarriage.

It is important to note if the embryo was not viable due to a chromosomal abnormality for example, and a miscarriage was imminent, progesterone will naturally decline. Therefore it can be difficult to determine if a miscarriage took place due to a chromosomal abnormality, a progesterone issue or both.

THE IMPORTANCE OF THE FOLLICLE

There isn't a great deal of discussion about the follicle's influence on the developing egg, but its importance is immeasurable as the follicle is essentially where the egg grows up. Ignoring the follicle's importance in the egg's development is like ignoring how the environment we grow up in affects our growth and health.

Let's take a closer look at the follicle and the role it plays in fertility. Inside the follicle, follicular fluid is present. This follicular fluid surrounds the egg as it grows. The importance of this fluid and its relationship to the development of the egg has been recognized as far back as 1974 in the *Journal of Reproduction and Fertility*. Author R. G. Edwards writes, "The presence of follicular fluid in so many species testifies to its potential importance in ovarian physiology, including steroidogenesis (the making of hormones), growth of the follicle, ovulation, and maturation of the oocyte (the egg) as well as its transport to the oviduct" (fallopian tube).

It is also important to remember that after the follicle releases the egg, it must be healthy enough to continue progesterone production through the luteal phase (second half of the cycle) and also into the first trimester of a pregnancy. If follicular health is lacking, then doesn't it make sense that this could impact the health of the egg and subsequently the embryo, as well as the health and continual development of the endometrial lining?

Despite its significant contribution to the development of the egg and the endometrial lining, the follicle's importance is regularly ignored in mainstream medicine, but, thankfully, not in the laboratory.

A Stanford University study has shown that it can take eight menstrual cycles before the follicle ever appears on the ovary. Therefore, preparing the body to create healthy eggs from healthy follicles can take up to eight menstrual cycles. See the following diagram.

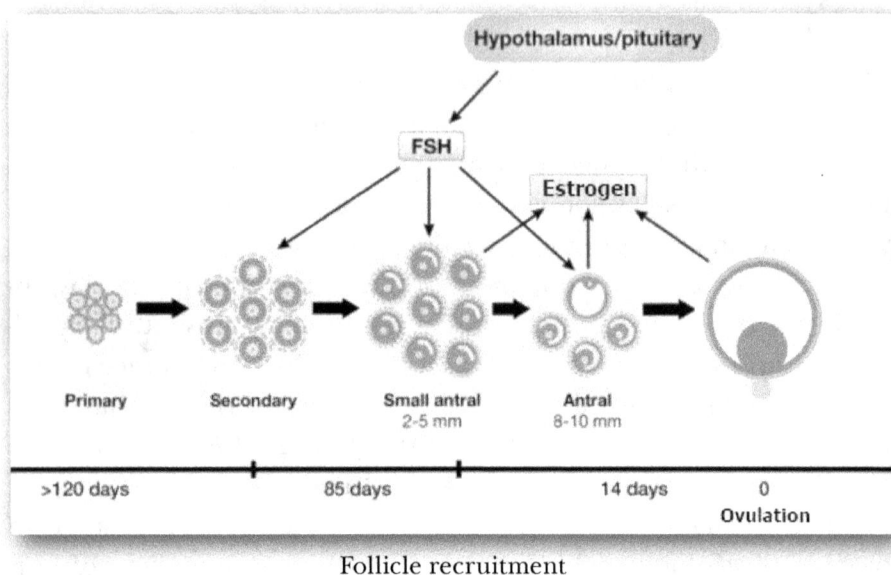

Follicle recruitment

At the clinic, on average, pregnancies tend to occur between six to eight months if dedicated to the program. Based on follicular development, and as you will read about very soon, sperm development, it is no wonder that pregnancies tend to occur six to eight months after beginning the program. Therefore, what you and your partner do consistently for six to eight months prior to becoming pregnant can impact the health of the eggs and the sperm. Many people are worried about a night of heavy drinking around ovulation but what is ultimately going to impact the health of the egg and the sperm are your consistent lifestyle choices and hormone balance throughout the six to eight months prior to conceiving.

Follicular fluid, the fluid inside the follicle, has been analyzed and found to contain many substances. They used to think that the fluid was sterile, meaning it has nothing in it, but in fact there are several important substances that influence the health of the egg. Antioxidants, bacteria, free radicals, hormones, minerals, glucose, enzymes, and toxins have been discovered in the follicular fluid.

Antioxidants present in the follicular fluid, for example, have been shown in several published studies in medical journals such as *Fertility and Sterility*. They discuss the importance of total antioxidant capacity in the follicular fluid being correlated with fertilization or pregnancies with IVF. This would likely be the case for natural pregnancies as well. In other words, the greater the antioxidant capacity of the follicular fluid, the greater the number of pregnancies in IVF.

This information helps to support why our Five-Step Fertility Solution which works toward optimizing cellular health and improving your antioxidant status and optimizing hormone balance, is beneficial for those wanting to conceive.

CHAPTER 4

DETERMINING OVULATION

MIKE AND TRICIA were both thirty-six years old when they decided to have a baby. After hearing and reading all the horror stories in the media and learning from their doctor that their time was running out, they decided to come to the clinic to prepare their bodies to create a healthy conception.

Nervously sitting in my consultation office, both admitted they did not have a clue when the best time was to have intercourse. Tricia had been on the pill for eleven years. They never gave ovulation a second thought. She had gone off the pill six months prior to our appointment, and it took three months for her period to come back. Because neither had been a fan of biology in school, Mike and Tricia felt a bit helpless in understanding what to look for and when to time intercourse. We discussed the basics of the female and male reproductive system. They hadn't realized how intricate these systems were, and their healthcare practitioner had not taken the time to explain to them what to look for regarding ovulation. Tricia reported that she was told by her doctor to "just relax, keep trying, keep having sex, and if it hasn't happened, come back in six months."

I showed Tricia and Mike what to look for when trying to detect ovulation, and they were pregnant within three months of timing intercourse.

Though it does not happen that easily with everyone, understanding when and if the female is ovulating is crucial to increasing your chances of becoming pregnant. Some couples have never had anyone show them when the best time to have intercourse is and how to figure that out. So many rely on information from the internet or apps on their phone but what one has to remember is many times these apps are inaccurate for a woman if she doesn't have a twenty-eight-day cycle every single month.

WHAT ARE THE SIGNS?

Ovulation, the time in a female's cycle when the egg is released, can be difficult to determine for some and very straightforward for others. This chapter is designed to help you understand that there are several different ways to determine ovulation.

When a female is ovulating regularly and even sometimes when ovulation is irregular, there are a few different ways to determine whether ovulation has occurred. Checking the following will help you in your quest to timing intercourse around ovulation and creating a viable pregnancy

- Cervical mucus
- Temperature charts
- LH surge testing via urine
- Ovulation tests using saliva
- Progesterone blood tests
- Ultrasound
- High-tech options to determine ovulation

CERVICAL MUCUS

One of the most common (and cheapest) ways women detect ovulation during their cycle is looking for the changes in cervical mucus. One popular and well known method among those in the reproductive world is the Billings Method, developed by Drs. Evelyn and James Billings. This method assists women to potentially track hormonal changes through their cycle by observing the changes in their cervical mucus and therefore determine ovulation.

The Billings Method discusses the following phases:

- Phase One: When menstruation ceases, the vagina tends to be dry—no mucus present. I have noticed that if there is discharge at this time, especially white or milky discharge that can't be related to intercourse the night before, it is often due to the female's diet (high in sugar and carbs) or she may not be processing those substances well in her system.
- Phase Two: Before ovulation, as estrogen begins to rise, clear sticky mucus can be noted.
- Phase Three: During the day of ovulation and sometimes surrounding days as well, the mucus tends to become more viscous, stringy, almost gel-like, similar to uncooked egg white. A woman may note that she can stretch the mucus a few centimeters (or an inch or so) between her fingers. Stretching of the mucus is not required to be fertile. It varies from individual to individual.
- Phase Four: After ovulation, the mucus decreases. If you are still having discharge, especially clear discharge, this could be a sign that estrogen and progesterone may be out of balance. If it is the white or milky discharge and not related to intercourse the night before, the comment above applies. Refer to step one of the Five-Step Fertility Solution: Optimal Eating Plan.
- Phase Five: A few days later, the mucus can become watery, and the vagina becomes dry again.

The consistency of the mucus matters because cervical mucus has been shown to support the sperm in their journey to the egg. The substances found in fertile mucus around ovulation can actually help improve the sperm's motility.

When you are timing intercourse around ovulation, it can sometimes be difficult to identify the mucus due to the semen that comes away after intercourse, and it's also true that excretions will change with arousal. Therefore, it is important to note that these mucus changes will vary from woman to woman. In the clinic, I have noted some women become pregnant when they have noticed only a minimal amount of mucus, and sometimes those with textbook mucus patterns continue to have difficulty becoming pregnant. Though mucus can be helpful for timing intercourse, it is a good idea to utilize ovulation-predictor kits, temperature charts, and, if needed, a series of blood tests to determine the levels of estrogen and LH to confirm the potential days of ovulation.

Billings Method

Advantage: If you only have noticeable mucus leading up to, at, and around ovulation, it can be a very accurate method of determining ovulation.

Disadvantage: If you tend to have different mucus throughout your cycle or are having intercourse frequently to conceive or just for fun, it can be difficult to determine the exact time of ovulation by mucus alone. Also, if you don't tend to have much mucus at all, the Billings method can be frustrating and confusing.

It is common for women to experience different types of discharge during their cycle. Usually discharge and mucus should only be seen leading up to or at ovulation. If a woman is experiencing discharge and not sure if it is normal this should be discussed with their health practitioner. Mucus/discharge can be used to track ovulation but if excessive and outside of the ovulation window, it may indicate an overgrowth that could impact conception or overall general health.

Here are some examples of mucus or discharge that women commonly experience and what it may mean.

✓ White discharge: White or creamy discharge accompanied by itchiness could be thrush or candida, that is, a fungal overgrowth that is oftentimes exacerbated or created due to excess high glycemic refined carbohydrates and sugar in the diet, not enough good fats and protein, or after the use of antibiotics. Some progesterone gels and suppositories used after embryo transfer with IVF can cause this as well. This is commonly referred to as a yeast infection or thrush.

If the thyroid is sluggish, you may also experience thrush even with very little sugar or refined carbs in the diet due to hypothyroidism being associated with decreased metabolism of glucose in the system. This glucose (think sugar) then feeds the overgrowth (potentially fungus or yeast) and the result can be the discharged discussed. Thick cottage cheese-like discharge could be Candida Albicans which is usually more extensive than thrush.

Sugar and refined carbohydrates are a person's worst enemy when trying to get rid of candida/thrush or a yeast infection. It is often necessary to go on a very strict eating plan for weeks to months to address the candida. See text box for suggestions to address Candida, thrush, or yeast infections.

⌒

Many people find the terms, thrush, candida, and yeast infection confusing, so let's take a moment to clear that up. They all indicate an overgrowth of a fungus, most commonly Candida albicans, which is a type of yeast. Thrush is a colloquial term referring to the white flecks that can be seen when Candida overgrowth is present. Apparently, thrush was supposed to refer to the color of the breast of the bird with the same name.

(Who knew?) A yeast or fungal "infection' is really an incorrect term. Technically this issue is not an infection but instead it is oftentimes an overgrowth of fungus or yeast that is already present in the body.

Under circumstances where our immune system is low, we have a high carb or sugar diet, or we are not metabolizing this sugar or glucose well in our diet for various reasons, we can end up with a fungal/yeast overgrowth, otherwise known as Candida or thrush

Some doctors will prescribe anti-fungal medications, many of which are not recommended in pregnancy. However the most effective way to address Candida is removing sugar and starchy carbohydrates from the diet. In addition, probiotics in the Lactobacillus family, inserted into the vaginal with a bit of coconut oil can help inoculate the vaginal flora and potentially decrease symptoms as long as this is accompanied by getting rid of sugars and high glycemic starchy carbohydrates.

Make sure the probiotic is from a reputable source (see step three of the Five-Step Fertility Solution) and mix with a tablespoon of coconut oil and apply once or twice a day.

Candida can be seen on the tongue, skin, genitals, and throat, or it can even be present in the blood if it is systemic.

✓ Yellowish discharge: Yellow discharge consistently accompanied by pain can be an indication of inflammation of the cervix, infection of the vulva (the opening of the vagina) and the vagina, but it could be a sign of sexually transmitted disease as well. When all of these have been ruled out, some health professionals theorize that yellow discharge could be remnant of the corpus luteum coming away, as well, since the corpus luteum tends to be yellowish in color. Oftentimes when it is not a medical issue and patients with this issue address their eating plan and utilize supplements such as probiotics, the yellowish discharge goes away. After intercourse at times, depending on the contents of the semen, the discharge may seem yellowish as part of the semen comes away with the discharge.

✓ Brown discharge: At the end of a period, old blood or brown discharge can be common, and this usually relates to less than optimal estrogen production and can be addressed utilizing herbs to help optimize estrogen balance. If brown discharge occurs at different times throughout the cycle, such as in the second half of the cycle and/or right before the period, its presence could be an indication of less than optimal balance between estrogen and progesterone. In some cases the brown discharged comes away around menstruation. This could be older blood that was trapped from the last cycle and as the new lining continues to develop, this old blood comes away. This is common but not a normal occurrence and optimizing hormone balance often clears up this issue.

✓ Greenish discharge: See physician to rule out possible infection.

✓ A physician should check odorous discharge of any color as this can be an indication of pelvic inflammatory disease (PID) or infection of the fallopian tubes, uterus, cervix, or vagina.

TEMPERATURE CHARTS

Whether you are new to or are an old pro with utilizing temperatures to determine ovulation or not, this section can give you an idea of how informative temperature charting can really be. Yes it can be frustrating for some but charting your temperature can be an effective tool to help you conceive.

Charting temperature to determine ovulation and to look at a woman's menstrual cycle over a period of time brings some women great stress because it reminds them that they are not pregnant, while to other women who are actively following the Five Step Fertility Solution, charting their temperatures brings hope and inspiration as they see their temperatures improving over time.

There are many nuances in a temperature chart that relate to how a woman's' temperature fluctuates through her menstrual cycle. In addition, the temperatures can indicate whether the thyroid and adrenals may be an issue for her.

Whether you consider temperature charting as your friend or foe, remember it is just information that can help your practitioner if they are adept at reading them and give you feedback about what maybe going on throughout your cycle. If done over a period of time, for many, it can be a great adjunct to determining ovulation.

Several women I have seen have saved the chart where their viable pregnancy was conceived as a keepsake to be included in the baby's book.

THE BIRTH OF TEMPERATURE CHARTING

The discovery that body temperature can determine ovulation began more than a century ago. Its connection to ovulation wasn't discovered until 1926, when a Dutch gynecologist named Theodoor Henrik van de Velde found that elevated temperatures extended beyond the menstrual cycle and made the connection of higher temperatures to ovulation. However, it was Kyusaku Ogino and Hermann Knauss who ultimately determined the ovulation period and timeline and who independently created the first calendar-rhythm method of birth control.

Temperature shifts eventually replaced the calendar-rhythm method because of the studies of Wilhelm Hillebrand, a German Catholic priest. Research continued through the 1960s, resulting in the analysis and interpretation of basal body temperature (BBT) charts. However, they were not deemed to be useful by couples planning or preventing pregnancy until 1983, when it was first taught to practitioners.

Research has expanded on how BBT can help determine ovulation and also assist in family planning. Known today as the Fertility

Awareness method by some, temperature charting is used to determine time of ovulation, along with several other charts and observations that follow cervical mucus changes and other fertility markers.

HOW TO ACCURATELY IDENTIFY OVULATION THROUGH TEMPERATURE CHARTING

As discussed, the temperature charting method has been used for years to help determine ovulation. Simple steps if consistently followed can reveal accurate ovulation times. The basal body temperature fluctuates as the hormones change in the body, but after the longest sleep, it is possible to get a reading of the basal body temperature without much interference, so in order to get the best reading, it is suggested to do the following.

- Use an oral digital thermometer (very difficult to read a mercury thermometer accurately without getting out of bed in the wee hours of the morning)
- Take your temperature after the longest sleep before getting out of bed.
- Some will take temperatures vaginally but I haven't found this to be necessary to obtain accurate readings.

For most people who work first and second shift taking temperatures in the morning gives the best data. If you are a shift worker, working different day and night shifts, the time you take your temperatures may vary. If a shift worker has gotten four to six hours of sleep, prior to reaching for the thermometer, temperatures tend to be more accurate.

Note: Fertility issues have been related to those who do shift work more often than those who work regular hours, so it is important to manage your sleep as best you can if you have no other option for your job.

One common reason patients avoid temperature charting is because they are told the temperature has to be done at exactly the same time every day. This is not necessarily true. As long as your sleep duration is relatively consistent, your temperatures can be accurate whether you take your temperature at the same time every day or not. The problem comes when you are sleeping much longer than usual (nine or ten hours and waking earlier and then staying in bed for a few hours) or less than four hours. If you have a strange temperature reading and you think it was because you got out of bed during the night, slept more or less than your normal six to eight hours, were sick, or indulged in a little too much alcohol the night before, make a note of that on your chart. One or two off temperatures in a month's time aren't going to make a big difference. If this occurs frequently around ovulation, however, it may be more challenging to determine ovulation for that month. That is another reason charting over several months will give you a better idea of ovulation and how you are progressing.

- Record temperatures on a temperature chart (see next diagram) or through an online service such as fertilityfriend.com.
- Record symptoms and changes of mood that you experience through your cycles, along with mucus changes. All of this information can give clues to what is going on with hormone fluctuation through the cycle and what can be addressed to optimize your health and fertility.
- The mucus changes can be recorded on the temperature chart to see if they indeed line up with what the temperature chart indicates as ovulation.

BALANCED TEMPERATURE CHART
Here is an example of what is considered a "normal" or balanced temperature chart.

Day of Cycle	1	2	3	4	5	6	7	8	9	10	11	12	13	14	15	16	17	18	19	20	21	22	23	24	25	26	27	28	29	30	31	32	33	34	35	36	37	38	39	40
Date																																								
Intercourse							O		O		O	O				O				O	O		O																	
Blooding	X	X	X	X	X																																			
Temperature																																								
99.5 F/37.5 C																																								
99.32 F/37.4 C																																								
99.14 F/37.3 C																																								
98.96 F/37.2 C																																								
98.78 F/37.1 C																																								
98.6 F/37 C																																								
98.42 F/36.9 C																																								
98.24 F/36.8 C																																								
98.06 F/36.7 C																																								
97.88 F/36.6 C																																								
97.7 F/36.5 C																																								
97.52 F/36.4 C																																								
97.34 F/36.3 C																																								
97.16 F/36.2 C																																								
96.98 F/36.1 C																																								
96.8 F/36 C																																								
How You Feel																																								

Balanced temperature chart

Keep in mind, balanced or normal does not always mean there aren't any issues. A temperature chart is simply one variable that can be used to monitor ovulation but even more importantly it is an objective way to monitor changes through the cycle when you are following the Five Step Fertility Solution. An experienced professional who has observed temperature charts over the years can show you how you are improving over time. When all you have ever seen is your own temperature chart compared to the "normal" temperature chart, it can be quite difficult to ascertain changes or improvements. You will however see a few tips about how you can evaluate your own charts based on the information in this section. I also have more information on my fertility membership website tipstogetpregnant.com if you are interested in even more detail about temperature charting, email thebabymaker@naturalfertility.com and ask for the temperature charting ebook.

SUSTAINED RISE: OVULATION

As discussed in the history of temperature charting, after ovulation occurs, a rise in temperature, otherwise known as a thermal shift, can be evident on the temperature chart. This thermal shift is preceded usually by a dip or drop in temperature. Presumably this dip or drop happens in the female to create an environment where the sperm are more likely to survive. Since the sperm are stored outside the body at cooler temperatures, the female's body accommodates by dropping in temperature around the time of ovulation to potential help the sperm survive.

Since there may be several drops in temperature in the follicular phase, it is important to note that ovulation is often not only determined by a drop in temperature but instead by a drop in temperature <u>followed by a sustained rise in temperature for four to five days or more.</u> This rise in temperature or thermal shift correlates with increasing progesterone production in the luteal phase, or the second half of the cycle. The leftover remnants of the follicle, that is, the corpus luteum, produces progesterone after it has released the egg.

Because the temperature rise after ovulation correlates with the female's progesterone production, this rise can give your practitioner a clue about the endometrial lining. It does not determine the thickness of the lining by any means or even the level of progesterone, but the rise and whether it sustains can signal to your practitioner whether progesterone support is needed to encourage a healthy lining. Adequate production of progesterone helps to ensure a healthy lining of the uterus, so a viable embryo has a good chance to implant. Signs such as a very light period or gradually diminishing flow after one day of normal flow could indicate an issue with progesterone production. In general, three days of moderate to heavy flow, then gradually tapering off to nothing over the following two days is generally accepted as a healthy period. However, everyone is different, and the menstrual flow should not be assessed on its own but as one factor in comparison to the several other factors discussed here. (The endometrial lining and the period flow can be significantly affected by stress, which will be discussed in our "Mind-Body" and "What Your Doctor May Not Have Told You about Your Fertility" sections).

The following is a very simple explanation of some different elements that can be picked up by temperature charts overall, besides just ovulation. As all charts can be different, it is important to talk with your practitioner trained in the Five-Step Fertility Solution about what your specific temperatures may indicate.

> ➤ Very low temperatures (96.8 degree Fahrenheit, or 36.0 degree Celsius, or below) can show possible issues with the thyroid or adrenals, both of which can affect estrogen metabolism and production or progesterone production. Prior to being able to use blood tests to diagnose, a thyroid disorder physician would use body temperatures as a guide. Dr. Broda Barnes, a physician born in 1906, showed the medical community the association between hypothyroidism and low body temperature. Dr. Barnes's research showed a correlation to low thyroid function and a temperature of 97.8 Fahrenheit (36.5 Celsius) or lower taken with a mercury thermometer in the armpit upon waking. Temperatures taken orally are usually lower than when taken in the armpit. A temperature at 96.8 degree Fahrenheit (36 degree Celsius) or below is often associated with a potentially sluggish thyroid when taken orally.
> ➤ Higher temperatures (above 98 degree Fahrenheit or 36.7 degree Celsius) at or before ovulation may indicate a more acidic environment or from the Chinese medicine perspective, too much heat, which could impact the survival of the sperm. Testing the pH of the urine in the morning and throughout the day can assess acidity in the system. In the morning, the pH should be about 6.2 and by midday 7.2.

If there appears to be an issue with acidity based on temperatures and urine pH, then working toward alkalizing the internal environment of the body is important.

There are alkalizing bottled water products on the market that can be found at most health food shops. I don't recommend these. I would rather see my patients eating foods that can naturally alkalize the system versus relying on a company to process water so that is is more alkaline. Instead, I prefer to recommend an organically-grown barley powder called Barley Life. This product has helped patients alkalize their system, and they have reported more energy while taking the powder and mixing it with a low glycemic juice and water or just water alone. If you are interested in this product, please e-mail info@ naturalfertility.com, and one of the staff members will send you information on how you can obtain this product for the wholesale price.

Higher or lower temperatures in some cases can also correlate with less than optimal thyroid and/or adrenal health, but additional assessments via blood tests and saliva tests would need to be done to confirm.

Should Men Chart Their Temperatures?
At times, women have asked me this question and the answer is yes, especially if there is a problem with the sperm count/and or a severe factor affecting two or more parameters of the semen analysis. It may also be beneficial if he is often complaining of fatigue or presents with a low libido. A man's temperatures will not fluctuate as much as a woman's temperatures. Men don't experience the hormonal changes that a woman does and therefore a significant thermal shift does not occur. But if temperatures are very low or very high, this can be a sign that support of adrenals and thyroid function may be needed. If the oral temperatures are out of the typical male basal body temperature range of 97.1 to 97.8 degree Fahrenheit (36.2—36.5 degree Celsius) upon waking on a daily basis, this supports further investigation and a program that supports thyroid and adrenal function to improve overall health and fertility. Because temperatures are relatively stable in men, I recommend recording his temperatures for seven to ten days a month instead of through the whole month.

As you can see, there is a lot to be gained by taking your temperatures. Temperatures are not just for ovulation anymore. Temperature charting can also give you and your practitioner clues about what to focus on to optimize your fertility. Some people do find this process frustrating. If this is you, please read through the next section about how to address the stress of temperature charting.

THE STRESS OF TEMPERATURE CHARTING

For some women who have been charting their temperatures for months and months, the process can be quite stressful.

Samantha told me that temperature charting was a constant reminder that she was not pregnant, and it was really getting her down. Her doctor also told her it was a waste of her time. I explained to Samantha that the temperature chart does not have to be perfect in order for a person to become pregnant, and it only gives an indication of what may be happening with hormone fluctuation. It does not tell a woman whether she can or cannot become pregnant. I have teenage girls, women in menopause and even men keeping temperature charts because it provides me with very useful information related to thyroid and adrenal health. I tried to tell Samantha that it was her perception of how she was thinking about temperature charting that was causing her stress, and I encouraged her to change that perception.

For some women, that little talk helps, and they change their perception about charting. They look at it as simply a tool to tell me a bit more about their body, but for women like Samantha, our conversation only helped for a few weeks and the stress and anxiety returned. Because temperature charting is so beneficial, I suggested a few different ways to keep track of temperatures that can remove or reduce the stress of temperature charting so you can continue to collect this very valuable data about your health and fertility.

1. Realize there is no perfect temperature.

   I have seen women with the most erratic, inconsistent charts where I thought "this is going to take a while" become pregnant within a few months of starting my program, even though their temperatures weren't textbook. Conversely women with "perfect" temperature charts have taken longer to conceive.

2. Do not try to analyze the temperature chart on your own.

   As mentioned, see out an experienced professional to explain your charts to you. Preferably, choose a professional who has completed my Fertility Mentoring Program. They have benefited by my experience with analyzing thousands of temperature charts in nearly two decades. (email thebabymakernetwork@naturalfertility.com)
   So many women come in very stressed, saying their chart looks horrible and they are really worried; but when I look at it, I think it looks fine and I can oftentimes even pick out some improvements over previous charts. When you are only looking at your chart in comparison to one "normal" example, you may be overly concerned about it not looking perfect when there is nothing wrong with the chart. Your temperature charts aren't going to tell you whether you can get pregnant or not. While looking at them with a trained eye, they will, however, give you clues as to what to focus on to improve your situation.

3. If temperature charting is really getting to you, ask your partner for help.

When you take your temperature in the morning with an oral digital thermometer, hand it over to your partner to look at and enter into your chart or ask them to write it down on a calendar or diary so you can enter it into a chart a day or two before your appointment wita practitioner who has completed my Fertility Mentoring Program. This will work even if your partner gets up at a different time than you do because oral digital thermometers typically hold that temperature in memory until the temperature is taken the next time. By pressing the button again, the last temperature taken usually comes up first. Test your particular thermometer to make sure this is true for you.

4. If you have been charting for months and months and it is getting a bit much, discuss your frustration with your practitioner and take a break.

If you tend to be like some of my patients who have had it with temperature charting but aren't willing to give their partner the responsibility of recording the temperatures or the partner doesn't want to be involved, then discuss with a practitioner about whether there are certain days when you can take a break or discuss taking a month off.

Some women decide not to chart during their period, but this can often be a very important part of the cycle to take your temperatures because menstruation places additional physiological stress on the system and can affect thyroid function, which may in turn show up as low temperatures. So if you are going to skip any days, skip the last few days before your period is due. If ovulation is determined, you know when your period is due; so a month or so of skipping the last few days before your period is not going to make a huge difference in the interpretation of your chart. Some women can't help themselves and have to chart those last few days of the cycle to see if they may be pregnant. But keep in mind that you always have a home pregnancy test that you can do instead of relying on temperatures this late in the cycle. The stress of seeing your temperature drop if not pregnant can lead to you feeling down or anxious. The only time I would avoid this strategy is if temperatures at the end of the cycle have been deemed important by your practitioner. He or she may want to see those temperatures to track improvements on that particular part of the cycle.

5. Take a longer break.

Finally, if you are at the end of your rope and the beeping of the thermometer makes you want to throw it out the window, take a few months off from charting and discuss this with your practitioner. Sometimes it is beneficial to take a break and resume when you are feeling stronger and less stressed.

OVULATION APPS: BEWARE! THE RESULTS CAN BE WRONG!

There are more and more apps on the market today geared toward trying to make it easier to time intercourse or even avoid pregnancy. Each has its own bells and whistles to get you to buy them. Some are free and some are paid, but *most* do not work to detect ovulation for women whose cycles are irregular or longer than the typical twenty-eight-day cycle.

The average cycle length many of them use to predict ovulation is completely *inaccurate* and not at all useful to you when you want to time intercourse to create a pregnancy. If your friends are using them to avoid a pregnancy, please make sure you share this information with them as well. These apps only work for those whose cycles are *always* regular.

When your cycle is irregular or sometimes longer or shorter than twenty-eight days, these apps can give you a false indication of when ovulation is occurring because they calculate the average cycle length often from a previous cycle. This can cause an inaccurate reading related to when ovulation occurs resulting in incorrectly timed intercourse.

The only website and app that I have found that gives relatively accurate readings (although their predictions are also off sometimes too due to irregular cycles) is fertilityfriend.com. This is probably the most reliable, but when cycles are not regular, it is always important to seek the advice of a health professional who has significant experience in deciphering your temperatures.

ADVANTAGES AND DISADVANTAGES OF TEMPERATURE CHARTING

ADVANTAGES
When done over a period of time, charting your temperature can be very valuable. See the following examples:

➤ Keeping track of temperatures can help identify a short luteal phase (second half of cycle) which is often a sign of less than optimal progesterone production and subsequently poor egg health. All of these can affect implantation of an embryo and its viability.
➤ Temperature charting can help identify a low basal body temperature which could be related to issues with the thyroid,

adrenals, or both. These systems can impact reproductive hormone balance.

➢ A woman can uncover less than optimal fluctuation of hormones in the follicular, luteal phase or both.

➢ Women often keep track of symptoms through their menstrual cycle while charting temperatures, and this tracking can help identify a pattern of symptoms that occur each menstrual cycle. Depending on where these symptoms are occurring in the cycle, this can give a practitioner, who is familiar with how the reproductive hormones fluctuate, valuable information to create an effective program.

➢ Charting can help women feel empowered because they are finally able to participate in assessing and improving their fertility. The chart shows how different things affect their cycle temperatures and changes can be seen over time to help assess improvement.

DISADVANTAGES

Though temperature charting can give good information, it does have some drawbacks.

Your temperature can be affected by the following:

➢ A fever
➢ Excessive alcohol consumption
➢ Interrupted sleep
➢ Getting out of bed before temperature is taken
➢ Sleeping on an electric blanket
➢ Ovulation can only be detected after the fact, not leading up to ovulation so unless you have regular cycles, it is difficult to ascertain with certainty exactly when ovulation would occur. This is why it is important to use temperature charting as only one part of a comprehensive program to address fertility issues.

WHAT IF I DON'T OVULATE OR DON'T HAVE A PERIOD?

Early in my career of supporting couples with fertility issues, Amy came to me because her doctor said there wasn't any way she could get pregnant without taking hormones to make her ovulate. Amy had felt horrible on the hormones and didn't want to continue.

When I asked her why the doctor said she needed hormones, Amy replied that she was diagnosed with polycystic ovaries and hadn't had a period since high school. She was now thirty-two.

Amy and I discussed that many of my patients who had not previously been menstruating began menstruating while on our herbal formula and following the Five-Step Fertility Solution. So I was confident that within six months Amy would begin menstruating again, like so many others had.

Six months came and went, and both Amy and I were despondent. We really thought she should be having a period by now. Amy was going to go back to the hormones in a few months to see if, now that she had been on the herbs, the hormones might be more effective.

I thought this was a good plan. But a week later, I received a phone call from Amy. She was spotting! We were both very excited! I asked Amy to send in her temperature chart to me so I could see what was happening.

Lo and behold, Amy was not going to get her period after all. She was pregnant! She and I were elated and a little confused. How could she have gotten pregnant if she wasn't ovulating? Well, she clearly ovulated once so maybe it just took that long for her body to kick into gear. We left it at that.

Amy came back to me for baby number two about eighteen months after she gave birth to her first child. We had her do her temperatures again, and on closer inspection, there actually was an ovulation pattern—a dip followed by a sustained rise (although the rise was not as high as most, nor for as long). I suggested that Amy and her husband time intercourse any time after her period finished when she noticed a dip in temperature and or if she saw clear mucus, had food cravings, increased libido or other symptoms she previously noted around ovulation.

It took four months and Amy was pregnant again using this method while following the Five-Step Fertility Solution.

What can everyone learn from Amy's story?

1) You can still ovulate, even if you aren't menstruating.
2) Even though temperature charts give signals of ovulation after the fact, if you have irregular cycles or no cycles, if you time intercourse around the dips in temperature, you may just be hitting ovulation.
3) Temperatures, along with other signs and symptomatology, can be very accurate ways of determining ovulation when observed over a period of time.

It is extremely important to understand that just like it is impossible to determine what fertility issue you may be experiencing based on one simple test, using one or two temperature charts to get an indication of ovulation or other issues that may be affecting your fertility is not accurate. It is only when a series of temperature charts are done over a period of time that a well-trained practitioner can use these to assess ovulation and much more. Remember charting temperatures is ONE piece of a challenging puzzle. More pieces are needed to get a clearer picture.

Some health professionals have said that taking temperatures is a waste of time because they are inconsistent. This is based on studies that involved physicians who don't normally look at temperature charts and after a short period of training were asked to assess charts and ovulation of one or a few cycles. The problem with these studies is that the physicians or practitioners were inexperienced with temperature charts, and as discussed it's necessary to see a series of charts to detect ovulation and learn more about the woman's cycle.

When done over a period of time, if performed correctly by the female, consistency will emerge, and though the charts may not be perfect, the information can be very valuable to a health professional who is accustomed to interpreting temperatures. The information obtained from temperature charting is only an indication of what is happening, and further testing such as ovulation tests, blood tests, and even saliva tests are necessary to get the full picture.

OVULATION-PREDICTOR KITS

So far, we have discussed determining ovulation using methods that are no-cost (checking your cervical mucus) and low-cost (temperature charting: one-time purchase of a digital thermometer). If you want to confirm ovulation because it is difficult for you to detect any cervical mucus or your temperature charts are not showing clear ovulation, it may be necessary to move on to other means or use these as a means to check the accuracy of the temperature charts and mucus.

At your local pharmacy, you will find a variety of options called ovulation-predictor kits (OPK). Each of them may be measuring something different to determine ovulation.

Normally they measure one or two of the following?

- LH surge via urine
- E3G via urine
- Estrogen via saliva

If you are not sure when your cycle is going to start because it is extremely irregular or nonexistent, using ovulation-predictor kits could be a very expensive. It would be necessary to buy test kit after test kit and keep testing for a positive which could be several days or weeks.

Instead when you experience irregular cycles, start with temperature charting along with checking cervical mucus to pin down ovulation. Work with a practitioner such as those educated in the BabyMaker Network familiar with the Five-Step Fertility Solution to monitor your cycle and improve cycle regularity. Then as you have more information to go on based on these methods, move on to the OPKs.

For those whose cycle is slightly irregular or generally regular, the methods discussed next are worth considering.

LH SURGE VIA URINE

Several companies have developed ovulation-predictor kits that measure the surge of LH (luteinizing hormone) in the urine. A surge of LH occurs when the egg is releasing at ovulation. These tests can be found at your local pharmacy.

If a female typically has a twenty-eight-day cycle, then start testing about day eleven or twelve for the LH surge, which for a twenty-eight-day cycle, should occur on day fourteen. If the cycle is usually longer or shorter than twenty-eight days, subtract fourteen from the usual length of the cycle to come up with approximate ovulation date and begin testing a few days before this. For example, if a female has a thirty-two-day cycle, then thirty-two minus fourteen is eighteen, which would make the eighteenth day of the cycle the suspected ovulation date. To confirm this with the ovulation-predictor kit for LH, begin testing on day fourteen or fifteen through day eighteen or nineteen to confirm ovulation.

ADVANTAGES AND DISADVANTAGES OF LH SURGE TESTING
Advantages:

-   Convenient low-to-moderate cost and accurate if you have relatively regular cycles and a strong LH surge.

Disadvantages:

- Can be costly if you have very irregular cycles
- Can be inaccurate if you have PCOS or any other issues where your LH surges at times other than ovulation
- Gives only a one or two day window to time intercourse

ESTROGEN TRACKING VIA URINE

Some home kits can track estrogen in the urine, as well as the LH surge.

Estrogen or the byproducts of estrogen called EGS appear in the urine and give an indication that ovulation is approaching. They give a larger window to time intercourse versus trying to time intercourse on the exact day of ovulation.

Studies show that having intercourse one to five days before suspected ovulation can also yield a pregnancy. The sperm can live for up to two to four days in the uterus, waiting for a signal that the egg has been released.

Remember to read the instructions and information on each OPK so you know exactly what hormones you are tracking and how these relate to ovulation.

ADVANTAGES AND DISADVANTAGES FOR ESTROGEN TRACKING

Advantages:

- Gives a larger window to time intercourse—can be three days prior to the LH surge when the egg is released. This helps you know when to start increasing the frequency of intercourse.
- Low-to-moderate cost if you have regular cycles

Disadvantages:

- If you have irregular cycles and have no idea when ovulation is likely coming in, testing over and over can be costly.
- If your estrogen levels are on the low side and this is contributing to your fertility issues, you may not get a strong indication of ovulation approaching, and you may incorrectly assume you are not ovulating.*
- If you have high estrogen levels, you may have a continuous positive throughout your cycle, which is unrelated to ovulation.*

*Blood tests of estrogen, specifically estradiol, on day two or three and seven days after ovulation in comparison to progesterone, as well as a hormone called Sex Hormone Binding Globulin (SHBG), will help you determine if estrogen levels are higher or lower than normal. Elevated SHBG can mean elevated estrogen storage in the system; low SHBG can mean low estrogen, and in females, glucose metabolism issues including those with PCOS.

SALIVA KITS

Saliva test kits, such as the Maybe Baby, which are available in Australia, New Zealand and the UK, are another way to determine estrogen surge preceding ovulation. These tests are also useful to uncover issues related to estrogen fluctuation in the follicular phase.

Some women complain that these kits do not work well because they are not getting the resulting "fern" pattern indicated in the instructions, which signals upcoming ovulation. However, information such as this can be helpful for your practitioner because it may be a sign that estrogen is not surging optimally, which could be related to the fertility issues. The Maybe Baby can then be used to monitor improvements in estrogen fluctuations leading up to ovulation as the patient continues through a program such as the Five-Step Fertility Solution™.

Other companies can test estrogen via saliva without the apparatus the Maybe Baby offers; however, these companies can take days or weeks to send the results back so would not be beneficial for someone trying to time intercourse with ovulation. The Maybe Baby gives immediate feedback to the user.

ADVANTAGES AND DISADVANTAGES OF TESTING ESTROGEN IN SALIVA:
Advantages

- One time purchase of the apparatus (moderate price).
- Gives immediate feedback and a larger fertile window than only LH surge testing.

Disadvantages

- Some women find it difficult to get a clear reading.
- If estrogen levels are high throughout the follicular phase, the fertile window will be too long.
- If estrogen levels are too low, there may be no reading, even though the user may still ovulate according to blood tests for LH and progesterone.
- Available only in certain countries

BLOOD TESTS

These next few tests are a bit more invasive and may require seeing a physician or paying for them out of pocket, but they can be good indicators of ovulation to either support what has been detected via temperature charts and mucus changes. If ovulation is too difficult to detect using other means discussed, doctors will use blood tests to track hormone fluctuation leading up to ovulation. This can be stressful if cycles are typically long due to the amount of times you would need to have blood drawn but can be useful for those who have regular or relatively regular cycle lengths.

PROGESTERONE BLOOD TEST: DAY 21

The most common blood test to determine if a woman has ovulated is progesterone. Typically, this test is done on the twenty-first day of the cycle. A progesterone reading above 30 nmol/L or 9 ng/ml indicates that ovulation has taken place. This can determine if there was ovulation; however, one progesterone test on a specific day of the cycle is not a good indicator of WHEN ovulation took place. A single day-twenty-one test with progesterone over 30 nmol/L or 9 ng/ml can confirm that a female has ovulated but not when she has ovulated. This is where temperature charting and cervical mucus tracking can help narrow down the fertile window and pinpoint probable ovulation.

Advantages:

For women with regular twenty eight day cycles, the day twenty one progesterone test can be very accurate in determining ovulation if her luteal phase is 14 days. Simply subtracting fourteen from twenty one gives you the ovulation date. I still suggest temperature charts and observing mucus changes however to make sure the luteal phase is not longer or shorter than the average fourteen days.

Disadvantages:

Not Accurate for Irregular Cycles

Some healthcare professionals will automatically ask for a day twenty-one test for progesterone without knowing the length of the person's cycle. Therefore, if a female typically has a long cycle, that is, over thirty-four days or a varied cycle length, a day twenty-one test may not detect a progesterone increase because that person has not ovulated yet. For example, if a female has a thirty-six-day cycle, ovulation would usually be fourteen days prior. If fourteen is subtracted from thirty-six, this equals twenty-two, the day where ovulation should have taken place. Therefore, a day twenty-one test would not indicate an increase in progesterone, and the patient would be lead to think (incorrectly) that she wasn't ovulating and be offered treatment that she doesn't need and create unnecessary stress about having an ovulation disorder that she actually doesn't have.

DAY TWENTY-ONE IS *NOT* ACCURATE FOR WOMEN WITH IRREGULAR CYCLES

Progesterone tests should be done seven days after ovulation as this is when progesterone should be at its peak.

A test seven days after suspected ovulation can also give your healthcare professional an idea of the balance of the hormones progesterone and estrogen at that time of the cycle if estradiol is tested as well. The balance between these two hormones is important in detecting issues that may be affecting a female's fertility. More on this will be discussed in the chapter entitled "What Your Doctor May Not Have Told You about Your Fertility."

Progesterone is used regularly to determine if a person has ovulated; however, a progesterone test by itself does not give any indication of when the person ovulated. Seven days after ovulation is the best time for the test and other means of determining possible ovulation, such as ovulation-predictor kits, awareness of mucus, and temperature charting. Using all or some of these together can help identify the best time to test for progesterone.

TESTING ESTROGEN AND LH

Estradiol, one of many estrogens in the body, is associated with fertility. Estradiol begins to rise several days prior to ovulation. LH does as well, but LH has a larger spike or surge right at ovulation. Therefore, a series of tests starting three to four days before suspected ovulation can track the surge of estradiol and LH to determine with good accuracy whether a person is going to ovulate and approximately what day they have ovulated. This accompanied with an ultrasound to see if a follicle has released an egg can be very accurate. If a female is expected to ovulate on day fourteen, blood tests would be done every day or every other day from day ten or eleven, and the ultrasound would be done after suspected ovulation.

Advantages:

-   Works well for cycles that are regular or slightly irregular (one month twenty-eight days; next month thirty-two days, etc.).
-   Gives a wider window to time intercourse effectively

Disadvantages:

-   Not cost effective or realistic for very irregular cycles
-   Can be cumbersome and expensive to have blood drawn for several days in a row

ULTRASOUND

Many times, ultrasounds are done in conjunction with blood tests. An internal ultrasound can track the development of the follicles on the ovaries. A follicle is a good size and likely close to releasing an egg when it has grown to 18 mm or larger.

Tracking the development of the follicle while monitoring the LH surge and estradiol levels is a very accurate way to determine within a day when ovulation is happening. A drop in the hormones LH and estradiol after the rise, as well as the presence of the ruptured corpus luteum or ruptured follicle on the ovary, are indications that ovulation has occurred.

Advantages:

- Works well for cycles that are regular or slightly irregular (one month twenty-eight days; next month thirty-two days, etc.)
- Gives a wider window to time intercourse effectively
- Extremely accurate when accompanied by blood tests

Disadvantages:

- Not cost effective or realistic for very irregular cycles
- For anyone who works outside the home, it can be challenging to have blood drawn for several days in a row
- Repeated ultrasounds and blood tests can be very expensive

In the past it has been difficult to document the exact time an egg was released, but gynecologist Jacques Donnez took the only known pictures of an egg actually being released from the follicle while doing a partial hysterectomy on a forty-five-year-old woman (and they say forty-five-year-olds don't have any eggs!).

The article and pictures can be found at: http://www.daily-mail.co.uk/health/article-1025956/Pictured-The-moment-human-eggemerged-ovary.html.

It was thought that an egg was released from the ovary suddenly, but the process documented by Donnez took fifteen minutes. It was also noted that the egg was surrounded by supporting cells that likely give it some protection as it enters the fallopian tube where fertilization usually takes place.

Though there are many ways to determine ovulation, at times, it can be difficult, depending on the particular situation. Women experiencing amenorrhea (absence of periods), irregular cycles, and less than optimal hormone balance may find detecting ovulation to be difficult. We discussed when to time intercourse with temperature charts if you aren't having a regular cycle or no period at all. Read further and you will find further suggestions through this book.

HIGH-TECH OVULATION-PREDICTOR DEVICES

Just as technology plays a role in our lives, work, and health, it has found a role in fertility. This section will cover these devices and provide information on their effectiveness.

THE DUOFERTILITY® MONITOR

Made by Cambridge Temperature Concepts Ltd., the DuoFertility Monitor (www.duofertility.com) is a relatively new electronic device that has been used since 2009 to assist couples in determining when they are the most fertile. Through a sensor that is worn by the individual, this monitor measures several components during sleep, including temperature, heat flow, and movement. The resulting information ascertains the quality of the individual's sleep and the best time to test basal body temperature (BBT). While thousands of measurements are taken during each night, the results are summarized, making it less complicated to interpret the results. The reasoning behind the many measurements is that continuous temperatures may provide more significant information than a single temperature taken upon awakening. Because the device is worn every night, it also eliminates the need for a woman to remember to take her temperature every day and at a consistent time. Studies have shown that the DuoFertility Monitor provides accurate results that are comparable to results received from performing transvaginal or internal ultrasounds. This device is available in the UK and soon to be available in the United States.

A bit expensive at 359.00 pounds for a three-month plan, it may be worth it to not have to do other testing such as blood testing to determine ovulation.

YONO Smart Earplugs

A new device, launched in August, 2015, by Yono Labs in California, is a smart earplug, worn in the ear to help women determine their cycles and identify when they are most fertile. YONO measures BBT in the ear through a small, silicone-covered thermometer. One advantage is that the ear canal is a closed environment that is not affected by room or external temperatures. Measuring temperatures between 70 and 120 times each night, these smart earplugs use this data to determine a woman's lowest resting temperature. The information is then analyzed and joined with information input by the user to predict ovulation. An app is used to communicate and store this information and help the user track their temperature and other symptoms monitored to indicate fertile periods and ovulation. Again, because this device also takes numerous temperatures throughout the night or resting period, it is believed that it can provide more accurate information than a single temperature taken in the morning upon awakening. www.yonolabs.com 149.00 USD.

These are relatively new devices, so as always search for reviews both on Google and the app stores to determine if these are devices you would like to purchase._I personally have not had experience with

DuoFertility or The YONO Smart Earplugs and therefore cannot vouch for their performance. As technology improves there will be more and more devices available to help those wanting to become pregnant and those who want to avoid pregnancy to do so without invasive tests.

CHAPTER 5

MALE-FERTILITY BASICS

MIKE CAME TO the clinic because he hadn't been producing sperm at all, though he had previously created a viable pregnancy with his former partner six years earlier.

Everyone was baffled when he and his partner Michelle weren't getting pregnant. Michelle had a regular cycle and two children with her previous husband. Test upon test showed that Michelle's hormone levels were still quite balanced at thirty-nine years of age, and she was ovulating regularly. It was not until we suggested that Mike be tested that the couple found out there was no live sperm present in his semen analysis. There were many sperm present but none of them were alive.

Needless to say, they were both shocked. How could this be? He already fathered a child. Upon further examination into Mike's history and current job situation, it was noted that he had been working around petrol in his job as a truck driver over the last four years. It appeared that the gradual increase in exposure to this chemical might have impacted his ability to create live, healthy sperm.

Within eight months of applying the Five-Step Fertility Solution™, Mike started producing live sperm again. There was enough sperm present to go onto IVF, and Michelle became pregnant on their first attempt together. Prior to applying the five steps, doctors had said they would need to have donor sperm to conceive.

Once pregnant with IVF, Mike and Michelle were over the moon but not quite as much as when they found out eight months after their IVF baby was born that Michelle was pregnant again. This time, it was a natural pregnancy.

MALE FERTILITY IGNORED

One of the most often overlooked areas when dealing with reproductive issues is the male side of the equation. It seems that if the sperm number is good, if they can swim, and if there are some normally-formed sperm, then all is right in the world of male fertility.

However, the sperm, like the eggs, are cells and depend on many factors to be healthy. Like the eggs, the sperm grow up in and around fluid (the testicular fluid) and are transported in the semen to the female reproductive tract through intercourse. Both the testicular fluid and the semen contain nutrients including antioxidants, as well as hormones, bacteria, toxins, enzymes, and even glucose and fructose (sugars).

ALL THE BITS AND PIECES ADD UP

So many times in a couple's situation, the male is ignored and only one or two preliminary tests are done to see if he has any issues. However, I can't tell you how many times pregnancies mysteriously result when his end of the situation is addressed with the Five-Step Fertility Solution.

Take Jill for example; she had come to me to prepare for IVF. She was in her early thirties, and they had removed endometriosis a few years prior but she still hadn't gotten pregnant. So along with her tests, I asked her partner for permission to review his semen analysis. He proudly told me that his doctor told him he had "super sperm."

Upon looking at his results, I could see that he had almost 100 million sperm, which is great, but the motility (the swimming ability) was sluggish (slower), than the normal range, and the abnormal forms were high when compared to the optimal levels I prefer to see in the clinic.

I discussed this with Jill, and she said they weren't concerned because the doctor said it wasn't a big deal and, if it was an issue, IVF would fix it. The reason the doctor said they weren't conceiving was likely the health of her eggs, although there were no tests to prove there were any issues with her eggs.

After two years of going through IVF, utilizing the Five-Step Fertility Solution for a few months here and there, instead of the six to eight months recommended Jill wanted to start another cycle. Jill's partner Mitch whose semen analysis was less than optimal in a couple categories was thinking it was too soon both from a financial point of view and an emotional one. He made a deal that if he would participate in the program to work on the quality issues they noted, she would put off their next IVF cycle for six months.

He became serious about all five steps; his motility improved to above the suggested parameters and his abnormal forms also increased a few percentage points. Within those five months of their preparation for the next IVF cycle, they became pregnant naturally.

It never hurts to have both partners involved in optimizing their health. As a matter of fact, the worst thing that can happen to the person following the Five-Step Fertility Solution is that they become healthier.

So let's take a look the basics of the male reproductive system to fully understand that all the bits and pieces really do count. As you read this section, remember that every organ or structure discussed is made up of cells and keeping those cells healthy is imperative to maximizing their function.

MALE REPRODUCTIVE SYSTEM

Get ready to move to the next level regarding understanding the male reproductive system. Male Fertility 101…

Let's just jump right in!

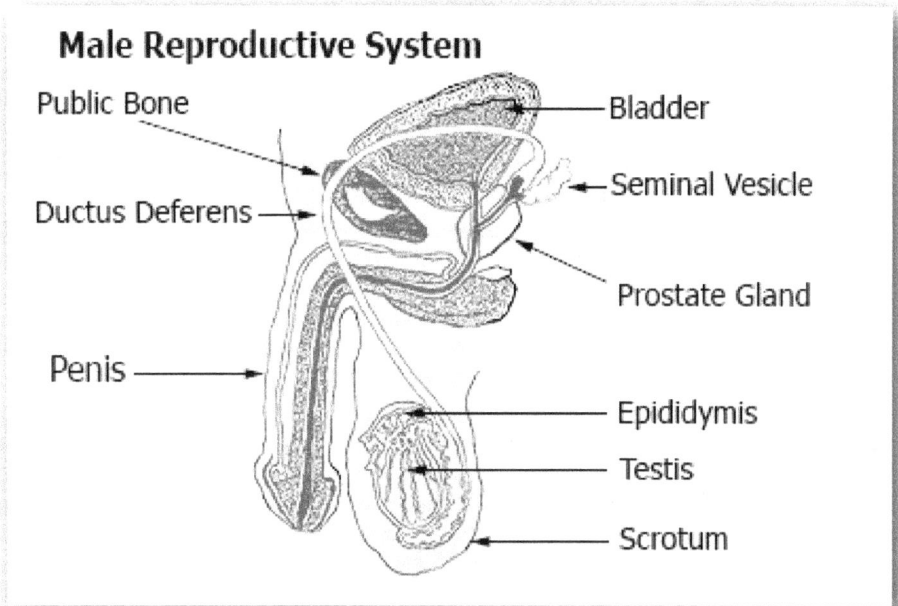

Male Reproductive System

Public Bone

Ductus Deferens

Penis

Bladder

Seminal Vesicle

Prostate Gland

Epididymis

Testis

Scrotum

Male reproductive system

Shortly before birth, the testicles (or testis as shown in the last diagram), the two small ball-like structures, will descend during fetal development to eventually drop outside the body and be contained in the sac called the scrotum.

Sperm are made in the testes in a number of small, tightly packed, fine tubes called seminiferous tubules. Between the seminiferous tubules, another type of cell exists, called the Leydig cells, which help produce the male sex hormone, testosterone.

Sperm production or spermatogenesis is a long and continuous process. Sperm are at different stages of their development in the testes at any given time. It takes about seventy to ninety days for sperm cells to develop into mature sperm. During this time, the sperm development depends on the nutrient status of the individual, this toxic load (what chemicals he may be exposed to and how his body is processing them, and his hormone production.

Environmental toxins have been shown to significantly interfere with this process. More on this in step two: Avoiding Endocrine Disruptors.

From each testicle, there is a long, highly-coiled tube called the epididymis that lies at the back of the testicle. The epididymis connects the seminiferous tubules to another single tube called the vas deferens.

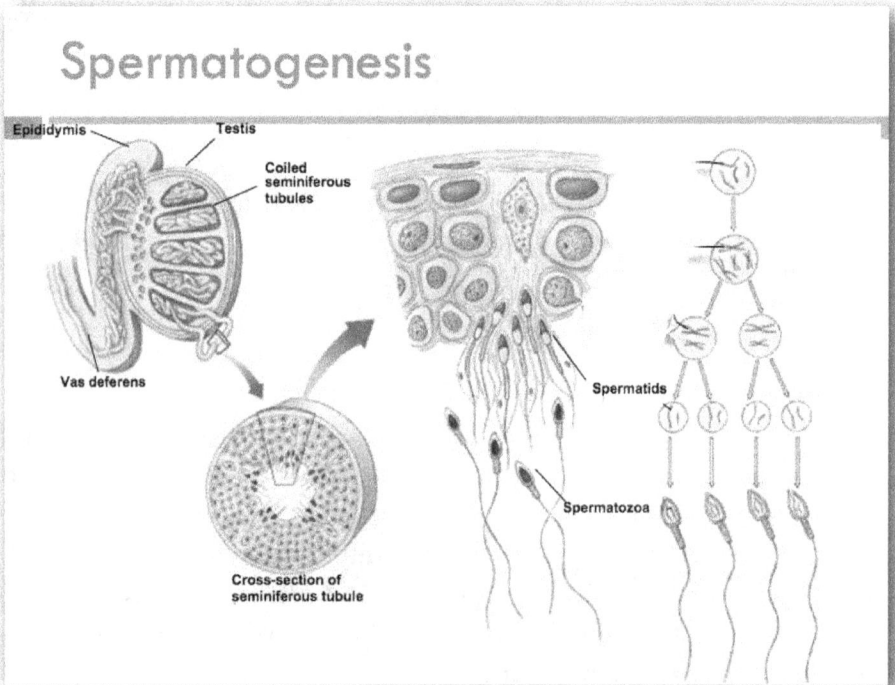

Spermatogenesis (The making of sperm)

After being released from the testes, sperm spend anywhere between two and ten days moving through the epididymis, where they become mature. It is during this process that the sperm undergo swimming lessons, so to speak, and develop their motility.

When ejaculation starts, the sperm travel from the epididymis via the vas deferens to the urethra (tube) in the penis, and the semen is added to the mix as they travel. The semen is not created in the testicles, but is released into the various tubes from the prostate, structures called seminal vesicles and another gland called Cowper's glands.

The semen contains nutrients, such as folic acid and zinc among others, immunosuppressants so the female's immune system doesn't attack the sperm, hormones, and unfortunately toxins (chemicals) that as you would imagine contribute to or take away from the health and swimming ability of the sperm

SPERM HEALTH AND DEVELOPMENT

How healthy sperm are created is similar to the development of any cell. Cellular health and development depends on many factors, such as nutrients available, the health of the cell membrane, to what degree toxins are present, and hormone balance.

Nutrients that we will discuss in step three of the Five-Step Fertility Solution are important to the sperm functioning and forming normally, as well as being able to swim well. In 2014 a review of clinical trials looking at the effects of oral antioxidants concluded that higher antioxidant intake was associated with higher sperm numbers, motility, and morphology (shape of the sperm).

When there is a male fertility issue, it is common for men and women to hear, "There is nothing you can do to improve the quantity or quality of the sperm." But reviews of research like the one above, several studies published in medical journals, and the clinical results I see support the fact that much can be done to improve their situation if they are willing to apply changes to their lifestyle, eating plan, and adhere to an effective supplementation program.

Manny was one example. He and his wife had been going through IVF for five years. They were creating embryos, but the embryos were either dying off early or not implanting. The doctors had used ICSI (Intracytoplasmic Sperm Injection), where one sperm is chosen by a scientist for each egg to be fertilized. The lack of implantation was said to be due to Manny's wife and her age. She was thirty-six.

When Manny came to see us, he was amazed that there was evidence that some issues with the sperm could be addressed because he had been told that there was no hope and ICSI with IVF was their only option. I explained that it was likely that IVF was needed due to the poor quality and very low count of between two and five million sperm. Normal is considered 15 million and the optimal levels for the clinic on average are fifty million. (More on optimal levels versus normal in a minute). Therefore even according to medical standards, his count was low and out of the normal range.

Manny agreed to take six months to work on his situation to prepare for IVF. The six months would allow the sperm to go through two rounds of regeneration and hopefully be healthier and, as a result, contribute to a healthier embryo. Within four months, I received a phone call that he and his wife were pregnant with twins from a natural conception. This was more than what we all had hoped for.

Manny followed our suggestions and programs to the letter, and when he was retested at three months (one month before the natural conception), there was a significant change in count bringing him up to just about normal and a large increase in motility. His rapid progressiveness, or best swimmers, improved from 15 percent to 50 percent, while the count improved by more than six times its original number to 16 million.

Manny's story illustrates three points:

1. Poor embryo development or lack of implantation is not always a female issue. The sperm's job does not stop after fertilization. The sperm contributes to the ongoing development

of the embryo. This has been shown in studies such as the one published in the medical journal *Human Reproduction* in 2014 titled "Paternal Influence of Sperm DNA Integrity on Early Embryo Development." Essentially this study shows that if early development of the embryo is lacking, it can be a factor with the sperm even when all sperm parameters appear to be normal.

2. ICSI may overcome the inability of the sperm to fertilize the egg, but it does not necessarily improve live-baby rates. If the sperm cannot fertilize the egg, it is not always a problem with the egg. There may be a critical issue with the sperm that is being ignored. There has been a huge increase in the number of ICSI cycles done with IVF, but this has not correlated with increased number of live births. One review of several studies on ICSI revealed it actually had no impact on whether a couple would create a viable embryo, that is, live birth. The rate of using ICSI has increased to 76 percent of cycles from 35 percent with no apparent benefit http://www.livescience. com/49507-ivf-icsi-procedure-increasing.html.

Researchers argue that ICSI makes IVF more expensive without any benefit and in most cases is not needed.

3. In many cases, a man can contribute to improvement in different areas related to his sperm with optimal nutrition, hormone balance, and lifestyle modification.

If a couple has not experienced a pregnancy without utilizing contraception for more than six months, it is always important to test the sperm through a semen analysis and other more detailed tests to determine whether there was any issue noted with the sperm from the tests.

THE SEMEN ANALYSIS

A man and woman both contribute to the health of an embryo and ongoing pregnancy. Therefore, when a couple experiences fertility issues, the preliminary investigation into a diagnosis or cause will include both the male and female most times. Typically but not always, that investigation includes diagnostic testing of the male's sperm. Many refer to this test as a sperm-count test; however, this semen analysis not only provides the number of sperm, but it also reveals whether the sperm have the expected shape (also referred to as sperm morphology), the percentage of the sperm that are swimming (known as motility), and how well the sperm are swimming (progressive, nonprogressive, immotile).

When the semen analysis comes back normal and doesn't identify any issues or significant abnormalities, the male is usually deemed to be healthy and not responsible for the inability to conceive. From that point, the attention is placed entirely on the female, who is subjected to more extensive testing in order to determine a cause and then treatment with drugs to attempt to control her reproductive system.

This is a good time to point out that "normal" is not always optimal for fertility. Science even supports this fact with some impressive findings. We'll discuss in greater details when normal is not optimal in fertility in the bonus section of this book. One such case that's related to male fertility and reproduction is the issue of sperm quality, not quantity.

TYPICAL SEMEN ANALYSIS NOT ENOUGH

Recent research has shown that the typical semen analysis does not analyze all the potential issues that could impact fertility. In fact, numerous studies have suggested that further testing is actually necessary. Unfortunately, it is rarely ever done.

That doesn't mean that additional tests have not been developed. Indeed, there have been some breakthroughs in the testing of sperm and semen that show a great deal of promise. One in particular is a genetic test that takes a look at the ribonucleic acid (RNA), which is a molecule that is highly concentrated in sperm cells and plays a role in fertilization and the development of an embryo.

A study lead by Dr. Stephen Krawetz in the journal of *Science Translational Medicine* reported that a test, which is scientifically referred to as next-generation sequencing of spermatozoal RNA, could provide answers that can help doctors determine the best and least-invasive fertility treatment, while saving the couple both time and money on testing and treatments. Unfortunately at this point, sequencing of spermatozoal RNA is not available to most couples, but the findings from this test are important to all couples where the male had a normal semen analysis.

Through next-generation sequencing, analysts can identify 648 RNA elements in a sperm cell, each of which contributes to a male's fertility. The study showed that sometimes sperm cells don't contain all of those elements—and the more elements that are missing, the less likely it is that natural, spontaneous conception will occur.

The results of this study are important because they reveal the need for increased testing in males, as well as potential issues that could impact a couple's fertility. First, it has been the standard practice that when a traditional sperm test does not reveal any issues, that is, the count is within normal parameters, a good percentage of the sperm are adept swimmers, and the sperm has the usual, expected shape, the focus on the ability to conceive is then placed on the woman. Yes, the sperm test did not indicate any problems—but there is one problem: the test focuses on the quantity of the sperm and their movement but not on the quality of the sperm.

ADDITIONAL OVERLOOKED TESTS
DNA Fragmentation: Often Overlooked Yet Extremely Significant

Studies into male fertility have brought enlightening news for couples who have difficulty achieving pregnancy. One of those tests that are available but rarely utilized delves into the DNA of the sperm, specifically sperm chromatin. A test called the Sperm Chromatin Structure Assay (SCSA) determines if a male's sperm has fragmented (or damaged) DNA which can affect whether an embryo continues to progress.

Here is how it works:

Chromatin, which consists of DNA and proteins, makes up the twenty-three chromosomes in the head of the sperm. The test, commonly referred to as the SCSA, identifies the existence of DNA fragmentation in the nucleus of the male's sperm. Results have shown that if more than 25 percent of the sperm are fragmented, there is a reduction in the likelihood of pregnancy. The optimal levels we see in the clinic are actually closer to less than 10–15 percent of sperm fragmentation.

What causes DNA fragmentation? There are many factors, including diet, disease, smoking, drug usage, age, excessive alcohol consumption, testicular temperature, pollution and other toxic exposure to chemicals. Many of these factors and their effect on fertility are discussed in detail in this book. Nearly every one of these factors can be addressed—with a bit of effort on the man's part.

DNA fragmentation testing tells us so much more than the traditional semen analysis. Remember, traditional testing only determines a male's sperm count and motility, but it doesn't give us many answers about the quality of the sperm. Therefore a basic semen analysis might not indicate issues that are likely to affect fertility. If a pregnancy doesn't occur within a year of trying, further investigation such as DNA fragmentation testing is warranted for the male even if he had a "normal" semen analysis.

Both the male and female should prepare their bodies for a healthy conception together. Remember, the months preceding conception determine the health of the egg and the sperm that gradually unite to create a viable pregnancy. Ignoring the male's health means the couple is ignoring 50 percent of the couple's fertility.

Is a Normal Semen Analysis Enough to Create a Viable Pregnancy?

Issues with sperm count and quality may mean that the sperm are unable to get to the egg to fertilize it, or in the case of a low count, there aren't enough sperm to be able to make the arduous journey to the fallopian tubes and fertilize the egg.

But what if the sperm is normal based on what is accepted as normal and seen on the semen analysis results. Is everything fine?

As discussed earlier, research now shows a semen analysis could be normal but there may be a problem with the DNA of the sperm. If too much of the DNA is fragmented, it often leads to miscarriage, slow growth of embryos, or no growth at all.

Why then do doctors just consider the *normal* on the semen analysis to be the definitive answer regarding whether there is a male fertility issue? I wish I had a good answer to that question, but the fact is, what doctors consider normal is not the number or percentage that the majority of men have on their semen analysis.

For example in table 1A the World Health Organization (WHO), the organization that sets the parameters for what is considered normal on a semen analysis. The following chart is based on the men's semen parameters whose partners became pregnant within twelve months of discontinuing contraceptive use.

The figures represent the following:

➢ Total count, not usually considered important on most semen analysis.

➢ Sperm concentration or density: Also referred to as count

➢ Motility: progressive and nonprogressive. This is represented as a percentage of the sperm that are swimming generally forward (progressive). Nonprogressive are sperm that are swimming but ultimately not making any ground. Think of them as swimming in circles or very slowly. Therefore nonprogressive sperm are thought to be less likely to make it to the egg.

> ➢ Immotile sperm: percentage of sperm that are not swimming at all.
> ➢ Vitality: percentage of sperm that are alive.
> ➢ Normal forms: percentage of sperm that are shaped normally. Abnormal sperm can have two heads, a crooked tale, two tales, abnormally shaped head, and so on.

Parameter (units)	N	Centile								
		2.5	5	10	25	50	75	90	95	97.5
Semen volume (ml)	1941	1.2	1.5	2.0	2.7	3.7	4.8	6.0	6.8	7.6
Total sperm number (10^6 per ejaculate)	1859	23	39	69	142	255	422	647	802	928
Sperm concentration (10^6 per ml)	1859	9	15	22	41	73	116	169	213	259
Total motility (PR+NP, %)	1781	34	40	45	53	61	69	75	78	81
Progressive motility (PR,%)	1780	28	32	39	47	55	62	69	72	75
Non-progressive motility (NP, %)	1778	1	1	2	3	5	9	15	18	22
Immotile spermatozoa (IM, %)	1863	19	22	25	31	39	46	54	59	65
Vitality (%)	428	53	58	64	72	79	84	88	91	92
Normal forms (%)	1851	3	4	5.5	9	15	24.5	36	44	48

Source: Cooper et al., 2009. WHO Manual, 5th edition, 2010

Table 1A WHO parameters

The columns 2.5 through 97.5 on the right are listed as centile, which is a fancy word for percentage. To explain this fully, let's take the sperm concentration, for example. Fifteen million is considered normal on most semen analysis today. But let's look at this a little closer via this table.

Find sperm concentration on the left hand side. Look to its right, and you will see the number fifteen. Follow that column up from sperm concentration of fifteen toward centile, and you see that fifteen million represents the fifth centile. But what does this mean exactly?

It means that fifteen million is the count or the concentration that 5 percent of the men exhibited who were able to create a pregnancy with their partner within twelve months of discontinuing contraception. OK, you might say, well what does that mean? It means that 95 percent of men who created a pregnancy with their partner had higher levels than fifteen million. Let me write that again: Ninety-five percent of men who with their partner created a pregnancy within twelve months of trying had *higher* levels than fifteen million. So why in the world would 15 million be considered *normal* when it is far from being even *average?* Another good question.

So what is an average sperm count and concentration? And why should we look at the average value? Well, the definition of average is "a number expressing the central or typical value in a set of data."

The average count would be the count or concentration based on the previous table representing the WHO parameters that are listed under the fiftieth centile. This value under the fiftieth centile would indicate 50 percent of men were able to create a pregnancy with their partner after twelve months of timed intercourse had less sperm, and 50 percent had more sperm. Therefore, this number represents the true average. And instead of the fifteen million which for some reason is considered *normal* we see that the average count is seventy-three million.

In other words, the average count for a man who has been able to create a pregnancy within twelve months of timed intercourse is seventy-three million, *not* the generally accepted normal range of fifteen million.

Motility is an important parameter to look at because it represents the swimming ability of the sperm. The more strong swimmers a male has should work in the couple's favor to increase the chance of a pregnancy because those sperm are more likely to not only get to the egg but fertilize it. It is the strength of the tail of the sperm and its ability to keep moving rapidly when the sperm meets the egg that enables the sperm to fertilize a healthy egg. Think of gridiron football and a running back who once he hits an object just keeps pumping his legs in the hope of getting just another yard or more on the field. If the sperm can continue pumping its tail fast and furious, it is going to have a better chance to penetrate the egg than a sperm with a tail that has less activity.

In table 1A, progressive motility for the fifth centile is thirty-two, so most semen analysis will list greater than thirty-two for the normal percentage of progressive motility to shoot for. But when we look at the fiftieth centile which represents the average number, we see that progressive motility should be above 55 percent.

Let's take one more example—normal forms of sperm. In table 1A normal forms are the last row in the WHO chart. The generally accepted normal for percentage of normally formed sperm is 4 percent of above. But again this is only the percentage for 5 percent of men who were able to create a pregnancy with their partner after twelve months. The average normal forms at the fiftieth centile is 15 percent.

I don't think it is a coincidence that the average sperm parameters that I see in the clinic when a pregnancy occurs are much closer to average numbers represented here in the chart from WHO, not the numbers accepted on the low side of the range as "normal".

Clinical averages from 2005 to 2015 (One thousand couples who became pregnant with a resultant live birth while participating in the program)

- Count/concentration > 55 million
- Total motility 55 percent
- Motility progressive > 50 percent
- Rapid progressives >50 percent These are the sperm that are swimming the fastest and most likely have a better chance of fertilizing the egg. WHO does not have a percentile for rapid progressives and therefore many IVF clinics do not measure it any more.
- Normal forms >6 up to 10 percent (strict criteria)

These are the parameters I suggest to patients to shoot for as we are working with men and or couples to improve their fertility. These aren't parameters that *must* be met in order to create a pregnancy naturally, but I have found that when the parameters are closer to the average while the male partner is participating in the Five-Step Fertility Solution, this increases the chances of pregnancy.

SIGNS THERE MAY BE FURTHER ISSUES WITH THE SPERM
How does a couple know when to suspect a potential issue with the sperm beyond a normal semen analysis or prior to having a semen analysis done?

Here are some signs that there may be an issue with the sperm and further investigation is warranted:

- No pregnancies from other long-term relationships where no contraception was used
- Family history of male fertility issues
- Chronic exposure to chemicals and toxins as a child or an adult. Adult farmers or children growing up on farms have an increased risk of chemical exposure.
- Occupational exposures: Exposed to chemicals on job currently or in the past
- Smoking marijuana
- Smoking cigarettes
- Other recreational drug use
- Use of testosterone or steroids: Use of testosterone has been shown to lower and in some cases completely eliminate spermatogenesis (the making of sperm)
- History of prostate issues
- Indication of prostate issues, that is, blood in the semen, stop starting while urinating, pressure with urination, or pain when starting to urinate
- Erectile dysfunction

- Pre-ejaculation
- Low libido
- Excessive fatigue
- Varicocele present in the testicle
- Small testicle(s)
- History of undescended testicles
- History of testicular torsion or other severe trauma to the testicles
- History of mumps
- Celiac disease

If any of these issues are present, then a semen analysis is warranted. If there is no pregnancy within six to twelve months of trying after ceasing contraception, then further investigation such as DNA fragmentation testing is strongly suggested.

If all parameters of semen analysis and DNA fragmentation testing appear to be normal, following the Five-Step Fertility Solution is a must to decrease inflammation and oxidative stress that could be affecting the sperm at a cellular level and unable to be assessed by current testing methods.

For blood tests recommended to further assess male fertility, please see the bonus chapter on "What Your Doctor Hasn't Told You about Your Fertility."

CHAPTER 6

TIMING OF INTERCOURSE

WHEW! YOU MADE it! Hope you were able to stay awake for the most of Reproduction 101. Now, onto the really interesting stuff and one of the most popular questions I hear from couples—when is the right time to have intercourse for baby making.

Intercourse: it has been called the "baby dance" on fertility forums and "making love" in relationships. And we all know there are other terms or phrases to describe it that I can't repeat here. But no matter what it is called, the fact is, many couples are misinformed about when it is the right time to have intercourse to conceive.

When is the best time to have sex? How many times should we "do it" around ovulation? Every day? Every other day? I can't tell you how many times I get asked these questions.

The following are four steps to consider:

NUMBER 1: AVOID ANALYSIS PARALYSIS AND HAVE SEX
I know it sounds crazy, but one of the most common reasons for a prolonged time to pregnancy is because people aren't having sex or they are having intercourse outside the fertile window. It is common after trying for a while to create a viable pregnancy for couples to get extremely frustrated. This frustration tends to lead to tension between the couple that can incidentally or coincidentally result in arguments around the time of ovulation. This, in turn, can result in not having intercourse at all around the most fertile times.

Dean described the time leading up to ovulation as intense. He felt like he was on the clock and had to perform at certain times.

Eventually, he lost interest in sex with his wife, Jo, and noticed that this extra pressure usually resulted in arguments with Jo, about various issues around the middle of the cycle. These arguments didn't even need to be related to fertility issues but could be about anything. "So avoiding sex because we were mad at each other just led to more frustration and disappointment when her period eventually rolled around again," said Dean, proving they did not have a pregnancy.

Sound familiar? This scenario is much different than before a couple was "trying," isn't it? So much time was devoted to trying *not* to become pregnant pre-baby making that it can become a real pain to perform at a moment's notice while trying to conceive. The act that is supposed to be spontaneous, fun, and intimate turns into a science project with little intimacy and more methodology.

It is not uncommon to have this type of scenario play out when dealing with fertility issues because when you have sex every month solely for baby-making purposes, it can become quite challenging when nothing is happening.

NUMBER 2: MAKE SEX MORE INTIMATE, BOTH DURING THE FERTILE TIME AND OUTSIDE OF THIS TIME

If you have been trying for any length of time, I am sure you have become aware that baby making can feel like a huge chore at times. When a pregnancy hasn't happened after months of trying, couples lose the spontaneity that used to precede intimate encounters. Once his wife became pregnant, one patient described what a lot of my patients confess to be thinking. He said to his wife after she found out they were pregnant, "This is great! Maybe now we can start making love again, instead of just trying to make a baby."

Dean and Jo could definitely relate to that statement, and after much discussion and noted frustration in many consultations, both Dean and his partner Jo finally laid it on the line and started communicating.

"I feel like a circus animal," he said. "I am expected to perform on cue. What happened to the spontaneity of it all? It used to be fun."

Jo, who felt like she had heard it all before, said while rolling her eyes, "Give me a break! I go through so much to try to make this happen. I am poked and prodded with needles and ultrasounds. I take pills to help me ovulate that make me physically ill. I have supplements coming out of my ears and take herbs to help. I run from doctor appointment to doctor appointment, and all I ask is for you to have sex at the right time. Is that too much to ask?"

As they sat in my office, sharing what was really bothering them, a light bulb seemed to go on for each of them. Dean, though he witnessed all the hoops that his partner was jumping through, never thought about how difficult and taxing this must be for her. Jo didn't realize Dean was feeling such pressure and couldn't understand why it was such a big deal. She thought he would be happy to have sex. When I asked when outside the fertile window they were having sex, they looked at each other and realized that they only attempted to have sex when she was ovulating, and it was quite an emotionless and often anticlimactic experience.

I had never realized how some men really felt about this until Dean opened up and said, "I am not an emotional guy, but what I realized in this process was that one way I did express my emotional connection to my wife was through intercourse. When the pressure was put on and it was more like we had to do it than wanting to make love to each other. I started to get angry and didn't really know why. Then we would only do it at once or twice a month, I felt really disconnected and pretty much felt like a sperm donor."

From this discussion, they vowed to do more activities together that didn't involve doctor's appointments and running to the pharmacy or chemist for more ovulation tests. They decided to revisit the reasons they married each other in the first place and focus on that, instead of just having sex to make a baby. Eventually, that resulted in more sex in the non-fertile time.

In addition, Jo agreed not to put so much verbal pressure on Dean; instead, she placed her temperature chart on the refrigerator and circled the days of probable ovulation. In that way, she or Dean could plan a more romantic evening around baby making. She stopped leaving ovulation sticks on the bathroom counter as a subtle reminder that it was "that time of the month" and also stopped announcing when he arrived home or texting him from work to "be ready." Instead Jo started sending him flirtatious texts at various times of the month just like they used to do when they were dating and early in their marriage. Dean started to do the same.

Texting may work for some couples and leaving ovulation sticks lying around the bathroom may annoy the heck out of another or be helpful. The point here is couples can develop their own system that works for them. Communication is key to working out what works.

Dean and Jo began focusing on what they liked about each other, instead of what they hated about the baby-making process, which helped them reconnect and eased the pressure a bit. When either one felt overwhelmed, they agreed to talk about it and plan together what their next step would be.

Improved communication can result in a better understanding of what your partner is going through. This can enhance the emotional intimacy in the relationship, and an increase in physical intimacy can follow, even outside of the ovulation window.

NUMBER 3: THE FERTILE WINDOW IS LONGER THAN YOU THINK
Now that we have established the importance of having sex and connecting through love making at times other than ovulation, it is important to understand the best times to have intercourse to create a pregnancy based on the research. Studies have shown that having intercourse up to five or six days before ovulation, leading up to ovulation, the day of ovulation, and one day after a positive ovulation test (or indication of ovulation per temperature chart) can create a pregnancy.

Though there is debate about how long the egg actually survives once released—some studies say twenty-four hours, and some predict only a few hours—it is confirmed that the sperm can survive within pockets in the uterus in cervical fluids for up to six days. It seems there is some kind of signaling that occurs once the egg is released, and sperm that were dormant in the uterus are noted to begin swimming again toward the fallopian tubes once the egg is released.

The recommendation, therefore, is to begin having intercourse up to five or six days before ovulation is predicted to occur. This may vary on whether there is an issue with the sperm, so continue to read for more info.

NUMBER 4: FREQUENCY OF INTERCOURSE
Some couples ask me if they should have intercourse every day or every other day around ovulation. Over the years, the advice from research has varied.

Based on data from couples at the clinic, when I see pregnancies, it appears that if there is no known issue with the sperm, that is, the sperm concentration is adequate (above 50 million/mL), overall motility is greater than 50 percent, and rapid progressives (best swimmers) are greater than 50 percent, and the normal forms of sperm are 6–10 percent, having intercourse every other day around ovulation appears to be fine. That means if ovulation is usually on day fourteen, then having intercourse on days ten, twelve, and fourteen is often adequate.

However, if there is a low sperm count or DNA fragmentation is noted in the sperm through further testing pregnancies appear to happen more frequently with more frequent intercourse, that is, every day around ovulation.

FREQUENCY OF INTERCOURSE DEPENDS ON THE SITUATION
There is also some speculation that sperm quality or quantity may be improved with abstaining from ejaculations three to five days prior to having intercourse around ovulation.

The theory behind this is to flush the tubes of the old sperm greater than five days before ovulation and then leading up to ovulation, allow sperm to build up for a few days before ejaculating again. Having intercourse every other day from four to six days before ovulation to the day of or day after ovulation appears to be most effective.

The lower the number of sperm and the poorer the quality, the fewer the number of days of abstinence recommended (unless giving a sample for a semen analysis). For example, if the sperm count tends to be low (less than 50 million/mL) and quality is poor, that is, motility less than 50 percent overall, less than 50 percent rapid progressives, or a very high percentage of abnormal sperm (over 96 percent abnormal or less than 4 percent normal), then I would suggest only one to three days of abstinence followed by frequent daily intercourse around ovulation.

For men with very low sperm concentration (concentration of 5 million/mL or less), another method has shown good results with some couples at the clinic. The theory behind this method is to create a buildup of sperm over a period of time to increase the concentration of sperm in the ejaculate. However, when I fully explain this method, at first, it is not often very popular among men, but it has been correlated with natural pregnancies in some couples where only a male fertility factor of oligozoospermia, or severely low count, has been given as a diagnosis.

In this method, (stay with me, guys) two to three days before expected ovulation, during intercourse the male orgasms but does not ejaculate. Most men look at me after I say this with an expression of "What the?" or "Huh?"

Yes. It can actually be done. Orgasm and ejaculation are actually two different events, although most often happen one right after another or appear to happen simultaneously. It certainly does take a bit of practice, per the men who have mastered it. The orgasm without ejaculation can be accomplished through masturbation alone or with intercourse. Again, the idea is to build up the sperm concentration closer to when the female is going to ovulate so there is more sperm in the ejaculate.

Still not sure about this?

Orgasm without ejaculation is also practiced in some forms of tantric sex originating in India. Since ejaculation in some of these circles is considered as the loss of life force energy, orgasm without ejaculation apparently allows the male to maintain his life force energy, and this can result in having sex for longer periods of time and even for the male and female both to be able to create multiple orgasms.

It is clear this technique is not for everyone. After going through relationship counseling with his partner, one man was told to cuddle his partner after sex to help satisfy her, so when I mentioned to him the possibility of trying to have an orgasm but not ejaculate, his first response was "Great, first I am told that I can't fall asleep straight after sex, and now you are telling me I can't ejaculate! What next?" After a few moments of awkward silence in my office, we all started laughing or maybe just his wife and I were laughing!

Finally, if DNA fragmentation of the sperm is present, studies have shown that frequent, daily sex appears to help decrease DNA fragmentation and increase the chance of conception. This correlates with findings from The American Society for Reproductive Medicine, which states that sperm health may actually be adversely affected if the male abstains from sex for more than five to ten days. (Penn State Hershey Medical Center article, "Infertility in Men."

DNA fragmentation of the sperm has also been related to the following:

- Miscarriage
- Poor early development of an embryo
- Unexplained fertility issues
- Reduced implantation rates

Reference: http://www.sciencedirect.com/science/article/pii/
S1110569013000137

⌇⁓

TIMING OF INTERCOURSE WHEN THERE IS NO CYCLE

Some women with ovulation disorders do not menstruate regularly or sometimes at all. Many of these women present with polycystic ovaries (PCOS), an issue that affects ovulation oftentimes related to insulin resistance (a state of prediabetes). PCOS is a multifaceted health issue that can be addressed and improved in many cases by using the Five-Step Fertility Solution. But other women have irregular or absent cycles without being diagnosed with polycystic ovaries, and timing of intercourse can be challenging for both groups when the cycle is irregular or absent.

If a woman has a regular cycle or it's only slightly irregular (a few days longer or shorter here or there occasionally), at least she still has a relatively reliable starting place to begin trying to determine ovulation using the tips in chapter 3, "Determining Ovulation." The woman with a very irregular cycle (every few months) or no period at all is often at a loss of what to do.

She is often told she is not ovulating at all because, according to blood tests, her progesterone levels never rise. Sometimes this is due to a blood test timing error as discussed in Chapter Four: Determining Ovulation. Many doctors recommend testing for ovulation via a blood test on day twenty-one without asking what the length of a woman's cycle is. As discussed day twenty-one is perfectly fine if the woman's cycle is twenty-eight days and she definitely ovulated on day fourteen. But if her cycle is longer than 34 days normally and the test was still done on day twenty-one, the test on day twenty-one will show she didn't ovulate at all when it is more likely she didn't ovulate yet. If her cycle has been pretty regular at thirty-four days, she will likely ovulate later (day 21 or later).

Also, we have had patients who have come to the clinic who have not had a period for years, and either begin having a period with the program or become pregnant before ever having a period. Yes, you read that right. They have become pregnant naturally without ever having a period.

Remember Amy? Her situation was discussed in Chapter Four, Determining Ovulation. Amy was not ovulating for years before she came to see me and still managed to have three children through the program without ever having a period.

Fiona had a similar case. She came to the clinic after not menstruating for three years. She had tried Clomid, which didn't work, and she felt IVF was not an option for her due to her finances.

While she was participating in our program, like most women with her history, i expected she would have a period within six months of starting. It just just a little longer than that. She had a period seven months after starting and subsequently became pregnant naturally.

Like Amy, Fiona was not able to gauge her ovulation by blood tests or urine tests. But after tracking her temperatures for a few months, we began to see the ovulatory pattern described in chapter 3, and she and her husband began timing intercourse around this pattern. In the seventh month, she started menstruating and subsequently became pregnant.

The doctor told Fiona that was probably the first time she ovulated in years. But whether she ovulated only that one time or had been ovulating all along, Fiona and her husband didn't really care. They are very happy with the two children they conceived while on my program.

The moral of that story is to find someone who has extensive experience in reading temperature charts, and go to them to help you analyze the temperature chart to see if there is possibly an ovulatory pattern that will be useful to determine the best possible times for ovulation and follow the suggestions regarding timing intercourse in chapter 3. Doing this, along with following the Five-Step Fertility Solution, can result in a cycle commencing and a much easier way of timing intercourse.

MYTHS ABOUT BABY MAKING

Fiona's and Amy's story busts some myths about baby making. For example people often say if you aren't having a period you are not ovulating but as we have seen from Fiona and Amy, that is not always the case.

Here are some other myths about Baby Making that have been busted.

1) There is no scientific evidence to support the idea that putting your legs in the air or propping up the pelvis with a pillow will help you get pregnant.
2) A woman should lie still after intercourse. There is some evidence that pregnancy rates increased slightly after Intrauterine Insemination (IUI) when women lay still for fifteen minutes following the procedure. The study showed 24 percent of women who lay still after IUI became pregnant while 18 percent of women who got up right away became pregnant.
3) A woman has to orgasm in order for the sperm to make it to the egg. Though theoretically it may help, a woman does not have to have an orgasm in order for the sperm to get to the egg.

Now that you know all about the male and female reproductive systems, how do determine ovulation, and when to time intercourse, let's move on to the most comprehensive system to help you create a viable pregnancy; The Five-Step Fertility Solution.

THE FIVE-STEP FERTILITY SOLUTION™

To Becoming Pregnant Naturally or with IVF

What You Can Do to Maximize Your Chances of Creating That Little Life You Long For...

CHAPTER 7

STEP ONE: OPTIMIZING YOUR EATING PLAN

FINDING YOUR FERTILE FOODS

THE RIGHT EATING plan is very important for a person who wants to create a viable pregnancy. When a male or female consistently adhere to a properly balanced eating plan like the one described in this chapter, nutrients will be more abundant, which can, help optimize the health of the cells of the reproductive system and throughout the body. Optimal amounts of nutrients can improve cellular health and hormone balance. Remember that the eggs, ovaries, follicles, endometrial lining, semen, and sperm are made up of cells whose function is dependent on nutrients as building blocks to aid in hormonal output and balance.

Following the eating plan outlined in this chapter can also decrease inflammation in your system naturally. Inflammation can be a barrier to nutrients becoming absorbed or utilized properly by the cells of the body and could impact the health of the reproductive system.

Imagine that a cell in your body is a house. In front of the house, there is a highway and across the highway are the nutrients and hormones that want to get into and act on the cell (house) to improve its structure and make the cell function better.

But on that highway in front of the house (cell), if there is a lot of traffic and congestion then it is going to be difficult for what is across the street to get to the house (cell). Some of that traffic can be inflammation. This inflammation can make it difficult for the nutrients and hormones to get the signal they need to get across the highway and into the house (cell: sperm, egg, etc.). Other things such as chemicals and other toxins can create issues on the highway as well. Those will be discussed in step two.

This step will help you clear the highway of much of the traffic and create a more optimal environment inside your body for the nutrients and hormones to get where they need to go and improve cellular health and function. This relates to all cells of the body, but specific to the reproductive system, we are working toward improving the health and function of the eggs, ovaries, endometrial lining, the semen, and sperm, all of which are cells.

Creating and following an optimal eating plan is the first step to helping men and women improve their fertility.

Sue and Mark came to us after five years of trying, and three of those years included several IVF procedures. They had created one natural pregnancy in between IVF cycles that ended up in a miscarriage at six weeks. Both were told to just keep going because their embryos looked good, and no reason had been identified for their inability to conceive; but money was running low, and they couldn't see how doing the same thing over and over again was going to yield a different result. At forty-one and forty-three years old, they felt beaten down by the system.

Blood tests for Sue's reproductive hormones showed a slight hormone imbalance between estrogen and progesterone, and through the IVF process, due to emotional eating and the stress of the IVF drugs on her body, Sue had gained over 12 kg or 26.5 lbs over the five years that they had been trying. Her triglycerides had gradually increased over time and had become slightly elevated. This can indicate insulin resistance, which contributes to inflammation and can be related to difficulty in becoming pregnant or maintaining a pregnancy. The good news is that this can be reversed for most people through changes to their eating plan.

Mark's semen analysis showed an above average count, good motility, but high abnormal forms, that is, 96 percent abnormal. Because sperm are cells, when there are high abnormal forms and all other parameters are normal, there can be an issue with the patient's eating plan and with digestion. Mark did complain of excessive flatulence (actually, Sue complained about Mark's excessive flatulence) and reflux, especially after alcohol consumption. This can lead to oxidative stress (will talk about soon) or lack of good bacteria in the gut and semen. All of this has been related to high levels of abnormal forms of sperm. So it is not surprising when adjustments are made to the eating plan and gut health we often see an increase in the normal forms of sperm. After working through an optimal eating plan for both Mark and Sue, we began to see the triglycerides coming down for Sue, and she lost 13 pounds (6 kg) over a three-month period. She felt much better and was able to begin exercising, which over the following three months helped her lose another 11 pounds (5 kg).

Mark struggled a bit with the change in his eating plan. Due to his occupation as a truck driver, he was used to eating out every day. This had included high glycemic carbohydrates, added sugar to his coffee six times a day, and a high amount of fried foods that contained trans fats and not much nutrition. After implementing changes, his new semen analysis showed an improvement of his abnormal forms (down to 92 percent from 96 percent with an even higher count), in addition to a loss of 17 ½ pounds (8 kg) over the first three months—he became more motivated to stick to a healthy eating plan. He was even motivated to do more exercise, so he washed his truck three times a week instead of once every two weeks.

Just as we were going to have Mark redo his semen analysis for a second time, six and one-half months after starting the program, it appeared that it wouldn't be necessary because Sue became pregnant naturally and ended up having a baby boy.

When they brought their little one in to meet me, Mark commented with tears in his eyes "I look at my son and can't believe he is ours. After so many years of trying, it seems unreal."

Sue added, "We really believe the changes to our diet and having the herbs helped us create our beautiful little boy. It still makes me a bit angry, though, that no one in the five years that we were trying before or ever during IVF had told us we needed to change our eating habits. Before coming to see you, I felt like I was drowning in a big black hole. I was gaining weight and felt like it was never going to happen for us, and with each failure at IVF, I was becoming more depressed and tired of it all."

While one of the facets of the programs at tipstogetpregnant.com and www.naturalfertility.com is herbal medicine, it is when people pay attention to step number one, two, three, four, *and* five that the magic really starts to happen. Seeing the look on their faces as they were holding their son...priceless.

The results of two studies were presented at the annual meeting of the American Society for Reproductive Medicine in 2011. Both studies strongly indicate a link between semen numbers and quality with nutrition.

Audrey Gaskins (Harvard School of Public Health) authored the first study, which revealed that diets rich in red meat and processed grains resulted in impairment of sperm's mobility. Diets rich in fish, fresh fruit, whole grains, and vegetables resulted in improved sperm motility, meaning a higher number of healthy sperm are moving around and, therefore, able to reach a woman's egg and contribute to conception.

The second study, which was conducted by Dr. Jorge Chavarro, assistant professor at Harvard School of Public Health, concentrated on sperm count rather than motility. That study showed that men who ate diets high in trans fat had lower amounts of sperm. In addition, the amount of trans fat actually showed up in increased numbers in both their sperm and semen.

While there are other factors that play a role in a male's sperm count and motility, these findings provide a strong association between a man's diet and the overall health of his sperm.

NUTRITION IMPORTANT FOR OPTIMIZING HORMONE BALANCE

In the Five-Step Fertility Solution, there is no single strict diet that everyone is given.

In the Five-Step Fertility Solution, there is no single strict diet that is given to every person. Optimizing a diet to optimize fertility is not a cookie-cutter process. There isn't a one-size-fits-all plan. Instead, it is better if your qualified health practitioner who is familiar with fertility issues has the opportunity to assess your eating plan and give you tools, possibly alongside a nutritionist who will optimize your nutritional intake. Instead of starting a whole new eating plan, if a person tweaks their current eating plan over time to make it more optimal, they are much more likely to stick to it in the long term.

Sim Wu knew her diet was poor and not healthy. Since moving from her native country as a child where fresh food was plentiful, because her parents struggled financially when she first moved here, she ended up growing up on cheap fast food in the Western world. She thought she was one of the lucky ones, though, because no matter what she ate, she never gained weight.

She and her husband had been trying for years to get pregnant, and she was put on a medication long term that was meant to keep her prolactin levels down. Unfortunately, this medication, when taken long term, also can contribute to depletion of progesterone in the system.

No one could tell Sim Wu why her prolactin levels were elevated; instead, she was just given a pill to keep them low. High prolactin levels, if you are not breastfeeding, are many times due to less than optimal thyroid function. Her physician had said her thyroid was fine, even though detailed tests of the thyroid were not performed.

Our first step was to have Sim Wu keep a food diary to assess what she was eating. On inspection of her food diary, we saw that Sim Lee's diet was high in trans fat, artificial sweeteners, high glycemic carbohydrates, and didn't include much healthy protein or good fats.

We went through the information that you will read in the rest of this chapter with Sim Wu, and after six months of a healthy eating plan, she came off her medication under her doctor's supervision. Her prolactin levels jumped up at first, but eventually after staying on the program and being monitored by her physician, the levels came down to a normal range. Four months later, she was pregnant with her daughter. She followed our Five-Step Fertility Solution™ and created an optimal eating plan and supplementation program that she felt she could maintain throughout her life. Not only was she happy about her pregnancy, but she also felt empowered that she could now contribute to raising her daughter on a healthy eating plan.

WHAT TO EAT: A SUMMARY

First, to ensure optimal cellular health, we want to make certain that you are consuming foods that create a well-balanced eating plan. In general, this includes a good balance of raw foods, whole foods, and some cooked foods that provide you with the balanced levels of low glycemic carbohydrates, proteins, and good fats.

LET'S START WITH CARBS, THE GLYCEMIC INDEX, AND GLYCEMIC LOAD
One of the first dietary factors we will ask you to consider is related to carbohydrate and sugar consumption. This is called the glycemic index and incorporates the glycemic load of a carbohydrate as well. The glycemic index represents a way for us to measure how quickly glucose (sugar) rises in the blood once carbohydrates (which turn into sugar) and sugars are consumed. When you eat a carbohydrate or have some sugar, glucose levels rise in the blood. Continuous and excessive rising and falling of glucose over days, months, or years can contribute to inflammation and, as discussed, impact the health of cells in the body.

Glycemic load takes the glycemic index into consideration but goes one step further. It includes the total amount of carbohydrates in the food you are consuming. So sometimes a food can be high GI (have a high glycemic index) but a low GL (have a low glycemic load).

So at first glance, a food that is high glycemic, like carrots and watermelon, might look like it could be an issue, but when you look at the carbs-to-water ratio, it is noted that the insulin response from this food is quite low, and therefore less likely to contribute to inflammation, unless that is all a person eats.

How It All Works

Your pancreas is an organ that releases a hormone called insulin into your bloodstream to keep the sugar (glucose) levels as balanced as possible. If your pancreas needs to put out significant levels of insulin at regular intervals to address excessive glucose (sugar) levels in your diet from sugars and high glycemic carbohydrates, this can lead to an imbalance of insulin, glucose, and fats in your bloodstream, which contributes to inflammation and stress on the system. In turn, this can affect hormone levels, and some people will go on to develop insulin resistance, the stage before developing diabetes.

Insulin resistance is correlated with inflammation in your body. This puts your body under stress and disrupts the optimal output of hormone including the hormones of the reproductive system. Insulin resistance has been correlated with fertility issues in some men and women. Insulin resistance is also prominent in polycystic ovaries. Recurrent miscarriage has been associated with insulin resistance, as well as difficulty becoming pregnant naturally or with IVF. If the eating plan is not changed, the next step after insulin resistance can be Type 2 diabetes. And the complications related to Type 2 Diabetes go well beyond impacting your fertility. People who develop Type 2 Diabetes can go on to develop high blood pressure, obesity, poor circulation and more severely blindness and amputations.

Eating foods with a low glycemic index (low GI) (less than fifty-five on the glycemic index scale) and low glycemic load (less than ten on the glycemic load sale) creates less of a rise in glucose levels and insulin levels. If there is an increase, it does occur more gradually, thus allowing the body to be able to handle the change more easily.

A good book to learn more about the glycemic index is *The New Glucose Revolution* by Jenny Brand-Miller. Alternatively, you can look at the website www.glycemicindex.com. Another great reference to learn more about how to optimize blood sugar and insulin levels through glycemic load and glycemic index of foods is Dr. Mark Hyman's excellent book called *The Blood Sugar Solution*. His website is www.thebloodsugarsolution.com.

CARBS AREN'T ALL BAD

Are all carbohydrates bad for you? Absolutely not. Carbohydrates contribute to creating energy and are a good source of short-term fuel our body needs. However, there are certain carbohydrates that can be detrimental to your health and too much of them can be detrimental to your fertility.

What kind of carbohydrates should you eat?

As discussed, start with low GI/GL carbohydrates, since these do not cause the huge rise in blood sugar and insulin that high glycemic and high glycemic load carbohydrates do. But this is only the first consideration. Eating low GI foods is great, but let's face it, chocolate cake can be low glycemic (low GI) as well. That is when understanding low glycemic load really comes in handy.

Common sense is the first intervention. Most people can look at a low GI chocolate cake and compare it to an apple that is low GI and know the answer to the question "Which one is more nutritious?" Go for nutritious the majority of the time because low GI chocolate cake has a moderate to high GL of twenty to twenty-two. A low GL is between one and ten; a moderate GL is eleven to nineteen; and a high GL is twenty or higher so common sense wins.

In other words, consider the likely nutrient content of the food or drink that you are consuming and use common sense. When it comes right down to it, to eat healthily, the vast majority of our carbohydrate consumption can be through vegetables and salads (five to six serves per day) and fruit (one to two pieces per day).

Many people complain or report that this eating plan removes all the sugar from their diet, but in actual fact, even low glycemic index and low glycemic load foods when they are carbohydrates turn into sugar in the body. When our eating plan is high in sugar and high glycemic carbohydrates, our taste changes. We tend to crave these foods more and healthier foods less. Removing these types of foods helps to change our palate to enjoying healthier foods. Michael Greger MD, FACLM states on his website Nutritionalfacts.org. The longer we eat healthier foods, the better they taste.

Remember, any carbohydrates turn into sugar. The key is choosing the right ones to support your fertility.

Here are some simple tips for a low GI/GL eating plan.

- Remove white flour products from your eating plan. Low GI/GL breads are spelt, sourdough, multigrain, and rye. (Note: If you are having gluten-free bread, make sure it is low GI/GL. Check the grams of sugar and shoot for as low as possible. Under 6 grams per slice would be ideal and no high fructose corn syrup, soy or other additives discussed in step two.)
- Significantly limit or completely eliminate packaged processed products. But on the odd occasion that you do buy something to make from a box, make sure it says it is low GI and check online to see if it is low GL. Keep in mind food from a box is processed and ultimately should be avoided or *not* be eaten regularly. Overall, consider whether the low GI/GL choice is a healthy one. For example, a low GI muffin versus an apple? I know you know the answer.
- Eat low GI fruits, such as apples, pears, peaches, nectarines, and berries, on their own for a snack.
- Eat higher GI/low GL fruits, such as melons and grapes, and high GI, Low GL veggies (carrots and beetroot) with a meal or other snacks that have protein or good fats. For example,

homemade coconut yogurt (protein/good fats) and fruit (carbohydrate/sugar) can be a nutritious healthy snack.

- If you are having white rice, choose a low GI rice, such as basmati or doongara rice or choose brown rice instead.
- Choose sweet potato or yams (low GI/Low GL) instead of white potato (high GI/mod GL).

FIBER AND WHOLE GRAINS

Fiber is an example of a carbohydrate that is very important part of the diet. It does an effective job of helping the body remove toxins efficiently and optimizing hormone levels by regulating bowel health. Fiber helps the fecal material (aka poop!) move through the digestive system appropriately, helping to create formed stools and compacting the stool so toxins are less likely to leach back into the system. Therefore, fiber can keep your colon healthy. Studies show that increased fiber intake is related to a decreased incidence of some cancers.

There are two forms of fiber, soluble and insoluble.

Soluble fiber sources include vegetables, fruit, oatmeal, and legumes of the type that partially dissolve in water. Insoluble fiber sources include whole grains, seeds, and the skin on fruits that pass through the digestive system mainly intact.

Legumes, psyllium and whole fruits (not fruit juices) are good sources of fiber and are a recommended addition to your eating plan. The juicing process of fruits removes most of the beneficial fiber, so keep in mind that if you are juicing fruits and vegetables, you also need to add fiber to your diet because juicing removes all the fiber. Adding seeds to your diet is also a good source of fiber

Diets that are higher in fiber help to slow the digestion rate and lead to better control of the glucose and insulin levels in your system, potentially decreasing inflammation and optimizing weight.

Note: Have you started eating fiber, and you're actually more consti-pated, bloated, or uncomfortable than you were before? This can be a sign that the bad bacteria in your gut is out of balance with the good bacteria in your gut. When this happens the bad bacteria are feeding off the fiber and are causing you to feel more bloated, constipated and uncomfortable. So if you are feeling this way with more fiber, then stop the fiber or decrease it while you add good probiotics or bacteria into the gut from fermented foods or probiotics. More about this in step three. After two to four weeks of probiotics support, as long as you have a good eating plan, you should see a difference in how you are tolerating fiber. You should actually feel fuller for longer *and* notice that you are emptying your bowels more completely.

MINIMIZE SUGAR INTAKE AND ELIMINATE ADDED SUGAR

Eliminating sugar (refined sugar) in the form of soft drinks, sodas, candy, and other high-sugar snacks (including diet drinks and sports drinks) is very important for your health and your fertility. When con-sumed consistently over a period of time, these highly concentrated sugary foods and drinks that have no nutrient capacity can negatively impact your health and fertility. This is not simply my opinion—in a study published by the *Journal of Epidemiology*, it was reported that soda drinkers showed reduced fertility.

Refined sugar contains no nutrients; it has no good fats, no pro-teins, no enzymes, or other helpful substances for our body. In addi-tion, calcium, magnesium, potassium, and sodium are depleted from the body when there is intake of excess sugar. These nutrients are essential for fertility and overall health.

Fertility issues are not the only health issue sugary foods and drinks are associated with; osteoporosis and other degenerative dis-eases can be attributed in part to depletion of nutrients from the system.

I see clinically when men and women remove sugar from their diet and limit the amount of high GI/GL food, the temperatures of both men and women often improve, hormone levels improve, and in some cases pregnancy results.

Maria, a thirty-nine-year-old lean female experiencing amenorrhea (absent period) due to polycystic ovaries, refused to get rid of the half teaspoon of sugar in her tea and coffee each day. She felt that she was not overweight, and, therefore, the "little bit of sugar" she was adding couldn't possibly be making a difference. I tried to explain that caffeine in coffee and black tea stimulates the adrenals—and along with the adrenal hormones such as cortisol and epinephrine that are released into the blood system, which are stimulants—so is glucose (which is basically sugar); therefore, any additional sugar significantly increases the glucose load and, in turn, increases glucose in the blood rapidly, contributing to a stress response in the body. Over time this can impact hormone levels..

Most of these beverages are consumed on their own or with a sugary snack. This elevates the blood sugar levels quickly, and insulin has to be dumped into the system quickly, too. This insulin dump makes the sugar levels drop quickly, and it makes you tired and sluggish thirty minutes to an hour or so later. Doing this over and over each day can result in fatigue and irritability, anxiety, and even depression, which is often associated with inflammation in the system and physiological stress on the body affecting hormone production.

After eight months on the program and still no period, Maria finally gave up the sugar in her coffee or tea. She did not begin menstruating, but two months later, she was pregnant.

"I can't believe it," she said. "I think that the program was able to work for me when I finally gave up the sugar. Unbelievable."

I can't say for a fact that her giving up sugar was the only reason she became pregnant, but it certainly seemed like too much of a coincidence and certainly in the long run if she keeps it out of her diet will likely improve her health. For women like Maria with polycystic ovaries (PCO), sugar is especially detrimental. Sugar is to women with PCO like Kryptonite is to Superman. It makes their system generally weak since women with PCO usually have issues with how their body metabolizes or uses glucose (sugar).

But whether a woman has been diagnosed with PCO or not, getting rid of added sugar can decrease inflammation and improve fertility.

Remove Artificial Sweeteners

Some people ask if they were to drink Coke, which is better: regular or diet? My answer is neither is a good or better option. Regular sodas can contain up to ten teaspoons or more of sugar in them, which significantly affects blood sugar levels. Diet sodas often contain artificial sweeteners, which are correlated with metabolic syndrome, weight gain, heart attack, and stroke. So in choosing between those two options, you best choice is *neither.* More discussion around sodas and soft drinks will be found in step two of the Five-Step Fertility Solution: Avoiding Endocrine Disruptors.

PROTEINS ARE OUR BUILDING BLOCKS

Proteins are essential for growth and repair. They play a crucial role in virtually all biological processes in the body. Keep in mind that many hormones are proteins!

Proteins can also provide a source of energy, and they are all low GI. Proteins help keep the sugar response low when a carbohydrate is ingested.

Generally, the body uses carbohydrates and fat for energy, but when there is excessive dietary protein or inadequate dietary fat and carbohydrates, protein is used for energy. If this happens too often and for prolonged periods, we can lose muscle mass; so if you are choosing unhealthy carbs and avoiding good fats, your body can eventually break down your muscles to create energy. This results in the wasting away of your muscle mass subsequent to inflammation and stress on the system, which, as we have already discussed, impacts your hormone levels and your fertility.

I see many articles online reporting that diets are often too high in protein. What I have noticed during the nearly two decades of reviewing food diaries, is not enough good protein for most people. Many people consume lots of processed and packaged carbs through the day and potentially don't consume protein until dinner. And if protein is consumed during the day, it is often from fast food or restaurants. People are also not eating healthy sources of protein from varied sources on a consistent basis. Many tend to limit themselves by only thinking of meat as protein.

⌒

If you are a meat eater, look for a butcher who sells grass-fed organic meat or at least hormone free grass-fed beef. Grain-fed beef can contain up to 50 percent saturated fat, while grass-fed beef contains approximately 10 percent.

⌒

It's important to consume adequate amounts of different proteins, which can be found in the following:

- Nuts (cashews seem to have a higher protein content than other nuts)
- Natural plain yogurt
- Chickpeas, beans, legumes (pulses)
- Fish

- Chicken, Pork, Turkey: (hormone free and certified organic if possible)
- Red meat: Grass-fed and lean
- Eggs
- Hard cheeses
- Peas
- Spinach
- Protein powders (whey and rice)

PROTEIN POWDERS

Protein powders are popular among those trying to lose weight and body builders. But can protein powders be beneficial for fertility? In some cases where time constraints make it difficult to prepare a meal, a protein drink with a clean protein powder is a good alternative.

Cow's' milk has two proteins: whey and casein. Whey protein is a popular ingredient for protein powders, whereas casein is more popular in protein powders for bodybuilders. Casein tends to be more difficult to digest on its own.

Casein also tends be inflammatory on its own, so to keep inflammation down, stay away from protein powders that contain casein. This is true for males and females. So if there is an ingredient on the list of a protein powder with the word casein in it, for example, calcium caseinate or any derivative of casein, then find another protein powder.

Some companies understand that casein has gotten some bad press per scientific studies and can hurt their sales, but instead of removing this ingredient from their formulations, they often list it as a name you wouldn't probably associate with casein, such as milk-protein solids or milk-protein concentrate. Avoid products with these types of ingredients as well.

Pea protein and rice proteins are a popular vegetable source of protein that does not expose you to the antibiotics and other medications that cows are subjected to, and in some people it is more easily digested. Pea protein, however, is not a complete protein like whey or rice, unless the pea protein is combined with rice milk. Rice protein, on the other hand, is a more complete protein than even whey protein.

Pea protein, rice protein, or whey protein powders can be made into a drink to accompany a meal or in a healthy smoothie form to substitute a good meal (recipes are available at the end of the chapter). These protein powders can also be sprinkled on a low glycemic cereal to add more protein to breakfast.

Based on a study in the 1960s, there is some misinformation about peas and fertility floating around the Internet. However, currently no recent studies have found an association with including peas in your diet and a decrease in fertility.

Newer products marketed for vegans as a ways to increase protein in their diet are on the market. Some contain protein from peas, hemp, chia, or chlorella, such as this product at http://proteinpowder.mercola.com/vegan-protein-powder.html. If you want to avoid animal protein and/or can't tolerate whey, that product is a good choice. Keep in mind that many vegetarian protein powders contain soy. Soy protein powders should be completely avoided.

SOY AND FERTILITY

Soy is also a source of protein, but I would not recommend any soy that is unfermented or not certified organic, especially while trying to conceive. I was skeptical at first that there would be an issue with soy and fertility, but after careful consideration of the independent research and observation of patients in my clinic, I began to notice certain hormonal changes through blood tests and patterns in temperature charts of those who regularly consumed unfermented soy, such as soymilk and western version of tofu.

Fermented certified organic soy, on the other hand, does not appear to have a negative impact on reproduction. This includes natto, tempeh, miso, and most soy sauces.

Asian countries eat much more soy than Western countries, but most of the soy they consume is fermented. In addition, studies in 2007 from Harvard Medical School, that were later published in 2008 in the medical journal *Human Reproduction,* showed a correlation between eating unfermented soy regularly and a lower sperm count. To read more on the truth about soy and why unfermented soy may not be as healthy as you thought, log into www.mercola.com and search for "The Truth about Soy."

I have seen an optimization of hormone levels with some clients after they go off unfermented soy such as soymilk and tofu, especially if it was a staple in their diet. Temperature charts normalized and hormone levels improved.

Some studies have also recommended making sure you are not feeding soy to babies and children because of possible negative consequences on brain development or pubertal development later in life.

GENETICALLY MODIFIED FOODS AND FERTILITY

The other issue with soy is over 94% of the soy grown in the United States is genetically modified or considered a genetically modified organism (GMO).

We have no idea how genetically modified crops will impact our health because tests on humans are scarce, but animal studies are not promising. According to GM expert Jeffery Smith, findings by Russian scientists discovered that GM soy effectively sterilized the third generation of hamsters that were fed the GM soy. In an interview with Dr. Joseph Mercola from mercola.com, Jeffery Smith shared the following:

One group of hamsters was fed a normal diet without any soy whatsoever, a second group was fed non-GMO soy, a third ate GM soy, and a fourth group ate an even higher amount of GM soy than the third.

Using the same GM soy produced in the United States, the hamsters and their offspring were fed their respective diets over a period of two years, during which time the researchers evaluated three generations of hamsters.

Unbelievably, the second generation of GM soy-fed hamsters had a death rate that was five times what the normal death rate was for the controls.

Worse yet, nearly all of the third generation hamsters were sterile! Only a single third-generation female hamster. Only *one* single third-generation female hamster gave birth to sixteen pups, and of those, one-fifth died.

Another bizarre side effect found in the GM soy-fed groups was an unusually high prevalence of an otherwise extremely rare phenomenon—hair growing inside the animals' mouths. Eeeck!

Unfortunately not all governments require labeling of genetically modified or GMO foods or ingredients. For example, unlike Australia, New Zealand, Europe, and the UK, the United States, despite growing support from a grassroots effort around the country, still sides with companies such as Monsanto that have a strong lobby against GMO labeling laws. Therefore, anything that is not certified organic when it comes to soy should be considered genetically modified.

Based on USDA survey data, genetically modified soybeans went from 17 percent of US soybean acreage in 1997 to 68 percent in 2001 and 94 percent in 2014, 2015, and 2016.

Speaking of GMO's, corn is another crop often genetically modified with 92% acreage dedicated to growing genetically modified corn in the USA (USDA stats). This includes popcorn kernels.

Therefore, I recommend to buy certified organic soy and corn if you are going to have them to decrease the chances that these foods may have a negative impact on your system.

GOOD AND BAD FATS

Fats are a significantly important part of an eating plan.

Your brain is sixty percent fat.

Our hormones come from fat.

And every cell in the body has an outer layer of fats and proteins called the cell membrane. The function of the cell membrane is to monitor what gets into and out of the cell. So you can see why fats are important to the body.

Despite the necessity of good fats in our eating plan to optimize our health, over the past two decades, the citizens of Australia, Europe, the UK, the United States, and other westernized countries have been brainwashed into thinking that *all* fats are bad for them. Therefore, this type of thinking has led to a host of low-fat and no-fat products in the market, which correlate with the rise of the obesity epidemic in the many westernized countries discussed. This could potentially be contributing to less than optimal fertility as well.

WHAT TYPE OF FAT IS GOOD FAT?

Now you understand why fats are an important part of optimizing your fertility and overall health, but choosing the right type of fat is most important. Good fats will not make you fat (unless you overeat) and good fats can even help you lose weight! A review of weight-loss programs showed that those that included nuts (a good source of fats and protein) had better compliance rates and showed more weight loss.

The right kinds of fat will help provide nutrition to your brain and every single one of the trillions of cells in your body, including the eggs and the sperm. A an eating plan too *low* in good fat can increase cholesterol, decrease fertility, and be associated with mood disorders such as depression or anxiety. Therefore it is important to eat the right type of fat to benefit your whole body, including the reproductive system.

Good sources of fat include the following:

- Raw nuts
- Avocados
- Olives
- Coconut
- Seeds
- Natural yogurts (Full fat, almonds (any nuts) or coconut based)
- Small fish (for more information on fish, see the section on toxins)

The wrong types of fat can lead to poor health, weight gain, and eventually chronic degenerative disease. For example, trans fats should be avoided completely. Trans fats are created by adding hydrogen to vegetable oil for the purpose of solidifying the liquid. They're found in partially hydrogenated oils (avoid if you see any derivative of this term on the food label) and are used as an ingredient in foods and baked goods.

Trans fats should be avoided at all costs. Did you know that trans fat basically turns into rancid fat when you eat it? Just imagine gulping down a spoonful of the grease after you make some bacon! That is essentially what you are doing when you eat food that contains trans fat.

TRANS FATS NOT GOOD FOR FERTILITY

Trans fats have been shown to affect fertility in several studies. A 2007 study from Harvard University revealed women who presented with ovulation disorders tended to consume more trans fat than their counterparts who ovulated regularly.

Governments around the world are beginning to respond to consumers' request that it should be mandatory for trans fat to be listed on the ingredients' label of all foods that contain it. I wouldn't however completely trust the labels that there is no trans fat in packaged or processed foods. Regulations in the United States allow a product that has less than .5 grams per serving or 2 percent trans fat to be labeled as zero trans fat products. Therefore, sticking to fresh foods and moving away from processed foods sold in plastics and boxes is the best way to completely avoid trans fat.

Around the world people and governments are taking notice. In 2007, New York City banned the use of trans fats in their restaurants. On a broader scale, in 2012, the US Food and Drug Administration (FDA) disclosed that partially hydrogenated oils were no longer "generally recognized as safe." In June, 2015, the FDA placed a total ban on the use or sale of partially hydrogenated oils and gave manufacturers three years to remove them from their products. (Source: http://www.fda.gov/ForConsumers/ConsumerUpdates/ucm372915.htm)

Dr. Steven Nissen, the chair of cardiovascular medicine at the Cleveland Clinic, elaborates on these findings.

"In the 1950s and '60s, we mistakenly told Americans that butter and eggs were bad for them and pushed people to margarine, which is basically trans fat. What we've learned now is that saturated fat is relatively neutral—it is the trans fat that is really harmful and we had made the dietary situation worse."

(Source: FDA Orders Food Manufacturers to Stop Using Trans Fat within Three Years, by Jen Christensen, June 16, 2015, http://www.cnn.com/2015/06/16/health/fda-trans-fat)

These are examples of foods that contain trans fat:

- Margarine
- Vegetable shortening
- Partially hydrogenated vegetable oil (look for these terms on the food labels)
- Deep-fried foods (high in bad fats in general)

- Many fast foods
- Most commercial baked goods (doughnuts, pastries, biscuits)
- Processed or packaged foods

I would suggest that you avoid these products and types of food for your overall health and your fertility, and especially for the health of any children you may have in your lives now and in the future. I know we are discussing fertility but you are trying to have children, so keep in mind heart disease is being discovered in children today, and one of the reasons is likely the poor, fat-ridden, sugary packaged food diet that has become the norm in many households. With all the high-convenience, low-nutrition food choices, it is important to take responsibility and take charge of what kind of fuel or nutrition you are putting in your body and the bodies of those in your family.

THE PERILS OF GROCERY SHOPPING

Now that you know everything you need to know about protein, carbohydrates, and fats and how they can impact your fertility, it is important to make this more practical.

How do you find the best products in the sea of choices that are found on the grocery shelves?

Did you know that according to the Food Marketing Institute, a trade association keeping track of food and marketing, the average grocery store in the United States in 2015 has over forty-two thousand products on its shelves? In 2008, the average number of products was just under nine thousand.

With this many products comes a vast variety of choices. Some of the more well-known brands of milk, for example, have more than eleven different varieties, and one brand of soup has over seventy different choices! When it comes to what products to buy, many Americans are overwhelmed by the sheer number of products and have difficulty knowing what to choose and what companies to trust.

Unfortunately, the way *most* people make their buying decision in the grocery store can be broken down into two categories. Based on the research from the International Food Information Council (IFIC), Americans choose their foods primarily based on the following factors:

1) Taste—96 percent
2) Price—73 percent

The IFIC's 2014 food survey revealed that more American consumers than ever before are basing their choices based on healthfulness. Seventy-one percent of consumers are choosing according to healthfulness in the 2014 survey, up from 61 percent in 2012.

But how are consumers determining healthfulness?

Most are relying on the media. But remember the media doesn't always reflect the truth, especially since the commercials, ads, and product placements people are bombarded with are not based on actual fact, but are paid for by the companies who have one thing on their mind, *profit*, not your health or your fertility. By law a publicly-traded company must first and foremost work toward producing profit for its shareholders, so decreasing costs and increasing sales are these companies' main objectives. Unfortunately, those factors don't often go along with helping consumers be healthy.

Companies spend *billions* of dollars marketing foods to children and adults. How is it possible to see through the fluff and spin of marketing campaigns and choose the best foods for your fertility and overall health?

It is time to discuss two key elements in choosing fertile foods that are great for your fertility now as well as your future family's health.

1) Navigate the grocery store to find the best buys for your health.
2) Read and understand food labels.

NAVIGATING THE GROCERY STORE

With so many options available to the average person—and because shopping can be very time consuming when reviewing every nutritional facts label—how can you make the process of buying healthy nutritional food easier? Preparation before going to the store and understanding the layout of your grocery store is the answer.

But before we get to the grocery store, the process starts before you leave the house.

First, don't go shopping when you're hungry—you'll have cravings and be tempted to splurge and buy more food, as well as food that provides low or no nutritional value.

Second, plan your menu and meals before you leave the house and purchase only the ingredients and foods that you'll need. Make a list and stick to it.

Now that you are ready to shop with a list in hand, whether you're altering your eating habits and creating a healthier eating plan or you're making changes to your eating plan to optimize pregnancy, the following tips will help you navigate the grocery store so you'll be more likely to purchase healthy, nutritional foods, and less likely to purchase processed foods that are high in sodium, sugar, and bad fats, a downfall of many shoppers when they choose convenience over health.

- Do the majority of your shopping on the perimeter of the store. Stay to the outer aisles, where you're likely to find the produce section for raw and fresh fruits and vegetables and the cold dairy section, where products like natural yogurt from milk or nuts, dairy products if you eat dairy, fish, and meats both white and red are usually displayed and kept cold.
- Avoid the center aisles of the store when you can; this is where most stores stock processed and prepackaged foods. It is also where most "junk" food, or food with little or no nutritional value, can be found.

- Processed foods that are high in sugar are often kept displayed in the middle of the shelves, making them easier to see. This prominent place is done for marketing purposes, and manufacturers often have to pay more to have their products displayed where they'll be seen easier and, thus, purchased more frequently.
- When possible choose fresh foods over prepared, canned or packaged foods.
- Beware of prepackaged dinners that are frozen since these can be very high in sodium. Avoid these when possible. Choose foods labeled low or no sodium. If you add salt to meals, you're better off adding it yourself with healthier options, such as Celtic or Himalayan salt. Regular table salt is made with man-made chemicals. Himalayan or Celtic salt contains natural trace minerals plus the sodium. A study published in the medical journal *The Lancet* in May of 2016 showed that those with too low sodium or high sodium levels in their system were at increased risk of high blood pressure and cardiovascular disease. A high-salt diet affected rats' puberty in a study at the University of Wyoming, but there is no definitive research about salt intake and fertility. The amount of sodium in a healthy eating plan appears to be between 3000 and 6000 mg per day.
- When purchasing frozen food, check the label for additives and preservatives, which extend the life, enhance flavor, or add color. Also, while some frozen food can be a healthy option, such as frozen vegetables, avoid those that are preseasoned or whole dinners and entrees that are prepared and packaged.
- Frozen fruits and veggies are a great option and in many cases have as much, and sometimes more, nutrient density than the fresh fruits and veggies in your fridge. Frozen fruits and some

veggies are also great for helping keep your healthy smoothies nice and cool.

- Learn where your favorite grocery store displays gluten-free products and other specially labeled products for specific dietary needs. Often, they are stocked separately from foods that do contain gluten. Note: Gluten-free processed products in packages are not always healthy and can be full of sugar. Choose whole foods that are naturally gluten free whenever possible if you have a low gluten or gluten-free eating plan.
- If the label or nearby advertising are geared toward attracting children or impulse buying (such as depicting cartoon characters), steer clear. Most times, these products are full of sugars or artificial sweeteners.
- Avoid the snack food, soda, pop and candy aisles. If you want to buy a treat once in awhile, buy a small dark chocolate bar versus a bag of cookies or snacks. You will tend to eat the small dark chocolate bar in smaller chunks, and it will last longer without the bag of plenty of snacks lying around tempting you at every turn.
- Avoid the bakery section and commercially baked products as these often contain loads of sugar and trans fat.
- When in doubt, purchase products with the least amount of ingredients. Make sure these ingredients do not contain long or difficult to pronounce chemical names.
- A quick glance at the ingredients listed on the label can tell you if there are artificial ingredients or additives. Restrict purchases of foods with artificial ingredients and ingredients you've never heard of or cannot pronounce.

DECODE CONFUSING FOOD LABELS

Now that you know the healthiest route around the grocery store, it is time to get educated on food labeling. It is best to have as much whole foods as humanly possible, but if it is not possible to make everything from scratch, it is important to be able to make the best choices you can regarding any premade or packaged foods that are purchased.

So when choosing these types of food, keep in mind that nation-wide analysis conducted by the Federation of American Societies for Experimental Biology (FASEB) found the amount of fat, sugar, and salt Americans are eating far exceeds the recommended limit. This is impacting the health of people in all westernized countries, and the low nutrient status and high artificial or natural additives could be impacting your fertility.

ENTER THE FOOD LABEL...

In 1990 in the United States, a law called the Nutritional Labeling and Education Act was passed, requiring all packaged foods to bear nutrition labeling. Food labels are a great addition to our shopping experience by providing information about the nutritional value of a particular food. In the United States, they are officially referred to as "Nutritional Facts" and can be found on the packaging of most prepared foods. While food labels are required in most countries, the information listed on them doesn't have to be preapproved before being sold. This means, essentially, manufacturers are on their honor to provide accurate information on their labels.

Nutritional facts contain some very valuable information, but only if you know how to read them, what they mean, and how the data relates to a healthy diet. To help you read and understand nutritional facts, a sample food label has been provided by the US Food and Drug Administration's website. It's important to note, however, that dietary guidelines change frequently, so the percentage (what is referred to as the percent daily value), serving size, and other information can and will change over time. It's also good to know that the information as it relates to one particular brand or product may be very different in another brand or product. For instance, the nutritional facts label provided is a sample of a typical macaroni and cheese dinner which of course would definitely NOT be a recommended meal for those trying to conceive. It is here for educational purposes only. The percentages, calories, and other information may be significantly different for a different brand of macaroni and cheese. Reading and understanding these nutritional facts will help you choose the foods that are healthiest and have the greatest nutritional value.

Sample label for
Macaroni & Cheese

Nutrition Facts

(1) Start Here ➡

Serving Size 1 cup (228g)
Servings Per Container 2

Amount Per Serving

(2) Check Calories

Calories 250   Calories from Fat 110

	% Daily Value*
Total Fat 12g	18%
Saturated Fat 3g	15%
Trans Fat 3g	
Cholesterol 30mg	10%
Sodium 470mg	20%
Total Carbohydrate 31g	10%
Dietary Fiber 0g	0%
Sugars 5g	
Protein 5g	

(3) Limit these Nutrients

(6) Quick Guide to % DV

• 5% or less is Low

• 20% or more is High

Vitamin A	4%
Vitamin C	2%
Calcium	20%
Iron	4%

(4) Get Enough of these Nutrients

* Percent Daily Values are based on a 2,000 calorie diet. Your Daily Values may be higher or lower depending on your calorie needs.

(5) Footnote

	Calories	2,000	2,500
Total Fat	Less than	65g	80g
Sat Fat	Less than	20g	25g
Cholesterol	Less than	300mg	300mg
Sodium	Less than	2,400mg	2,400mg
Total Carbohydrate		300g	375g
Dietary Fiber		25g	30g

Sample nutritional facts label (US Food and Drug Administration)

While the information in the food product label will vary, all labels contain specific categories that must be included. Let's review the information contained in the nutritional facts sample above, line by line.

SERVING SIZE

The serving size is based on the average 2,000 calorie (8,368 kilojoule) per day diet. All the nutritional information contained on the label pertains to one serving size. In the example above, that is one cup. Therefore, if you have two cups, you would also have to double the calories or kilojoules, percentages, and values listed on the label.

A package usually contains more than one serving size, and you will see how many serving sizes the package contains on the label near the serving size.

PERCENT (%) DAILY VALUE

This number reflects the percentage of nutrition or recommended allowance for this item in your daily diet. Again, this information is based on a 2,000 calorie (8,368 kj) per day diet.

CALORIES OR KILOJOULES:

The calorie category reveals the number of calories or kilojoules in one serving, based on the food in its present state. If you add any ingredients, spices, or sugars to the food before eating, it will affect the number of calories in each serving. Low calories do not always mean it is better for you, and remember the number of calories is related to *one* serving size. Some companies will make the serving size relatively small to make it seem like there are less calories or kilojoules per product.

As a subcategory, calories from fat reveals how many of the total calories from one serving come entirely from fat. Whether this is good or bad depends on the type and amount of fat, which are listed next.

TOTAL FAT

This is an important category because it tells you whether the fat contained in this food is healthy or one that should be avoided. First, the total fat is listed as a percentage value (the daily percentage value based on an average 2,000-calorie diet). For instance, if the total fat is 10 percent, that means that one serving of this food provides 10 percent of your total daily fat allowance for a 2,000-calorie a day diet. According to the Mayo Clinic, if you're on a 2,000-calorie-a-day diet, 400 to 700 calories can come from dietary fat, which translates to between 44 and 78 fat grams a day. (Source: http://www.mayoclinic. org/healthy-lifestyle/nutrition-and-healthy-eating/expert-answers/ fat-grams/faq-20058496)

Next, the total fat is broken down to reflect the type(s) of fat in the product. Typically, it will list saturated fats and trans fats. Avoid trans fat like the plague, and remember some countries, like the United States, allow a certain amount of trans fat in a product to be considered as zero trans fat, so whole foods once again seem to be a better choice.

Recently, saturated fat has been shown to be less threatening than once thought, especially when from sources like coconut, so reducing animal fat and increasing fats from nuts and seeds is a great choice.

For other good-fat choices, refer to the previous section discussing foods with healthy fats and those to avoid.

Cholesterol
Cholesterol content is next. The daily-value percentage is based on US FDA guidelines; however, persons with dietary restrictions or lifestyles should always use the dietary recommendations advised by their medical practitioner in determining their daily cholesterol intake.

Sodium
The main ingredient in salt, it is recommended that the average person keep their sodium intake to 3000–6000 mg per day. Less than 3000 mg and more than 6000 mg of sodium has been correlated with cardiovascular disease and high blood pressure. High blood pressure is a common symptom for women with polycystic ovaries (PCO).

Foods can be high in sodium even if they don't taste salty. Sodium is used to preserve food, extend its shelf life, add or enhance flavor, and is found in higher concentrations in many prepared, packaged, and canned foods.

TOTAL CARBOHYDRATES

Measured in grams, the total carbohydrates contained in food must be listed on the nutritional facts label. Then the total carbohydrates are broken down into three separate categories: sugar, starch, and dietary fiber. Keep in mind though that carbohydrates turn into sugar when ingested, and as discussed, not all carbs are bad. A balance of good low GI/GL carbohydrates are necessary in our diet, but too many of the wrong types of carbs, as discussed, can be fatal for your fertility.

Many studies discuss that a healthy eating plan should consist of 55–65 percent of the calories being carbohydrates. However, some experts find this to be too high of a level and feel it simply promotes weight gain. Dr. Mark Hyman recommends anywhere between 10 and 40 percent of an eating plan consisting of carbs, depending on whether you are trying to lose weight or maintain weight. I recommend 10–20 percent carbohydrate (50–100 g of carbohydrates per day) for weight loss. If you are trying to maintain weight and eat healthily, 20–40 percent is good to shoot for, which is 100–400 g of carbohydrate per day.

At the end of this paragraph is a helpful PDF you can download from Dr. Mark Hyman's book, *The Blood Sugar Solution,* which is an excellent source to help you optimize overall health. http://drhyman.com/wp-content/uploads/2015/06/Dr-Hymans-Carb-Intake-Recommendation-Chart-FINAL-copy.pdf

Dietary fiber: This is a subcategory of total carbohydrates. Look for foods that are high in fiber, which is listed in grams. Three to four grams per serving is good. Fiber helps to keep glucose from spiking. Increasing dietary fibers with foods higher in fiber is excellent.

Again, always choose whole foods high in fiber before the packaged variety. Remember, if you have difficulty with fiber, that is, you feel bloated or constipated after having fiber, your bad bacteria is too high in comparison to the good bacteria in your gut.

Starch: Although not mandatory, some manufacturers provide the amount of total carbohydrates that come from starch. Starch provides the body with energy, and it constitutes a portion of the calorie content per serving. One gram of starch is equivalent to four calories.

Sugar: Like starch, one gram of sugar also equals four calories. Processed and commercially prepared foods tend to be high in sugar as well as sodium. Use the sugar content found on the nutrition facts label to choose foods that are low in sugar, especially if you are reducing or eliminating refined sugar to optimize your health. Your total intake of sugar should be kept under 25 grams for the whole day. One teaspoon of sugar is 4 grams of sugar, and the World Health Organization recommends having no more than six teaspoons of sugar per day from all foods. The average American consumes over twenty-two teaspoons, or over 80 grams, of sugar a day, and the average Australian, thirty teaspoons or 120 grams per day. This isn't just added sugar, like putting sugar in a hot beverage. This is all the sugar consumed, that is, naturally in foods and added, per day.

PROTEIN

The body uses protein for energy and in the growth and metabolism processes. Each gram of protein constitutes four of the calories per serving. Too much protein can impact the health of the liver and kidneys, while a protein deficiency, usually caused by malnutrition, can result in weight loss (mostly muscle mass), impaired growth, and in extreme cases, serious illness. Too little protein affects our metabolism, our energy levels, and general performance.

The Food and Nutrition Board at the Institute of Medicine recommends, based on average weights, that an adult woman should be getting a minimum of 46 grams of protein a day (up to 71 grams if pregnant or breastfeeding). Adult men need a minimum of about 56 grams of protein a day.

I normally recommend up to 30–40% percent of the eating plan be related to protein. So 150–200 g of protein is where an average adult female or male on a 2,000-calorie eating plan can maintain a healthy weight.

Overall 20–30 percent good fat, 30–40 percent good carbs (unless trying to lose weight in which case increase good fats and decrease carbs), and 30–40 percent of good proteins.

VITAMINS

The nutritional facts label also provides vitamin information. This amount is listed as a percentage, as it relates to the total recommended intake of that vitamin on a daily basis to prevent diseases that result from nutritional deficiencies. The label will usually only list the specific vitamins in the food.

It is important to note that these nutritional facts are found on packaged products. Raw fruits, vegetables, and fish are often sold separately and are not prepackaged. They may not contain nutritional facts (particularly because there is no packing or label to affix the information to). However, prepared produce, such as salads, and lettuce, carrots, apples and other items that are sold by the package or bag may contain food labels for your reference.

GUIDELINES FOR A HEALTHY EATING PLAN

OK, you might be overwhelmed at this point and say, "Ugh! Just tell me what to eat and what not to eat." If so, here are some general guidelines to go by and some sample eating plans to go with the guidelines, as well. Hopefully, this will not only be your eating plan to increase your fertility, but your eating plan for a long healthy life.

- Eliminate white flour products and foods that contain them, such as muffins, biscuits, cakes, and so on.
- Eliminate white bread and wholemeal bread completely, and if you eat bread at all, limit this to one or two slices a day of multigrain, sourdough, or rye.
- Avoid anything that says "partially hydrogenated" or "hydrogenated."
- Avoid trans fats—margarines, vegetable shortening, partially hydrogenated vegetable oil, deep-fried chips, fast foods, and most commercially baked goods.
- Avoid low-fat and diet products as these usually have more sugar, unless they naturally are low in fat, such as lean meats. Two or more low-fat or no-fat products in the diet have been related to ovulation disorder in some women.
- Limit white rice to low glycemic brands, such as basmati rice. www.glycemicindex.com has a database which is helpful in sourcing low GI products.
- Brown rice is less processed so can be difficult to digest or breakdown for some. If it irritates your digestion, work on your gut health because this may be a sign of less than optimal levels of good bacteria.
- Limit fruit juices to only occasional use or avoid them as they are heavily concentrated and can cause a significant sugar and insulin response.
- Eliminate soft drinks, including diet drinks, which are full of sugar/sweeteners or chemicals. For example, a known carcinogen (cancer-causing chemical), benzene, has been found in some sodas, as have bromine or bromide—chemicals that have been shown to impede the absorption of important nutrients, such as iodine. Low iodine can significantly impact thyroid health, which in turn can affect male or female fertility.
- Diet drinks are often sweetened with artificial sweeteners such as aspartame or sucralose and should be avoided due to their

association with inflammation and weight gain. Funny how research has shown this to be the case yet companies are still allowed to advertise these products as "diet" products. This is true for "zero calorie," "zero sugar," or "naturally flavored" products as well. These products should be avoided.

- Significantly limit products with natural sweeteners such as stevia or xylitol. Though these products do not appear to impact blood sugar levels, any sweetener natural or synthetic has the potential to feed fungal and other yeast overgrowths such as Candida.

- Instead of adding sugar or sweetener to any hot drinks, use spices such as cinnamon to add flavor and improve blood sugar balance.

- Honey is high glycemic and has a high glycemic load therefore it should not be used regularly. However due to its antimicrobial activity it can be useful in hot tea such as lemon and ginger when you are experiencing a cough or a cold.

- Eat plenty of vegetables and salads. One large salad a day with five or six different veggies and salads (add protein as well) is an excellent source of carbohydrates for lunch or dinner when you add protein to keep the blood sugar levels regular.

- Eat one to two fruits a day. Fruits have fructose in them, which is sugar, but eating the actual fresh fruit versus the concentrated juices gives you fiber and wonderful antioxidants that improve your health. More than two pieces of fruit per day can be a bit too much sugar for some unless you are active and exercise frequently. The best time to have fruit is right after a workout. You can have a fruit smoothie with protein powder after a good workout to help with recovery.

- Apples, pears, and other low GI fruits are good to eat on their own, but make the effort to eat high GI fruits with foods that consist of good fat and protein. Some examples of high glycemic fruits are grapes, melons, mandarins and oranges

- High GI/low GL fresh fruits are, however, a good choice right after a workout when your body will be utilizing the sugar more quickly.
- Avoid fruit salads due to concentrated high glycemic fruit.
- Have one to two pieces of fruit a day.
- Eat grass-fed beef instead of grain-fed beef, and eat free-range chicken and free-range eggs with no antibiotics or hormones.
- Eat plenty of nuts and seeds, organic if possible, and one to two servings of small fish per week, such as whiting or sardines.
- Minimize gluten and investigate the possibility of celiac disease with your physician. Removing gluten completely has been a great benefit to the digestive health of patients. Improving nutrient absorption can then increase the nutrients that are able to get to your reproductive system, improving cellular health of the eggs, sperm, endometrial lining, and so on. Sticking to fresh food and avoiding wheat is a great way to start eating gluten free. If gluten free, remember to stick to whole foods that are naturally gluten free versus processed or baked foods that are listed as gluten free.

SAMPLE EATING PLANS/RECIPES

I am often asked, "What should I eat?" Patients often request a specific diet to follow when trying to conceive. A decade ago, I used to give a fertility diet to patients who came to the clinic, but I found that, with the exception of a few who followed it, most found it too restrictive because it was so different from their normal eating plan.

Due to this, I now ask patients to complete a food diary and gradually tweak their eating plan over time to help create a life-long realistic eating plan for them and their family. This accomplishes two things:

- Optimizes fertility in the short term
- Optimizes personal health and the health of the family for years to come

Remember, the worst thing that can happen on this program is that you get healthier.

EXAMPLES OF AN OPTIMAL EATING PLAN WITH PLENTY OF FERTILE FOODS

In this section I will give you some common suggestions that I have given patient about their food diary. But after applying the knowledge you learn here in The Baby Maker's Guide To Getting Pregnant you will likely be able to move beyond these suggestion and build your own healthy eating plan.

Eat meals that have a source of the following:

- Good protein
- Low glycemic carbohydrates (all carbohydrates turn into sugar when ingested)
- Good fats
- No added sugars (natural or artificial)
- Filtered water (preferable between meals) up to two liters a day.
- Gluten free if you experience flatulence, bloating, or heaviness in your abdomen after any meal and consistent fatigue after having gluten. Note other symptoms can be related to gluten sensitivity and gluten intolerance. The bestselling book *Wheat Belly* by Dr. William Davis is an excellent resource to discuss the issue with wheat and gluten in your eating plan.

EXAMPLES OF BREAKFAST

1. Two eggs, scrambled, poached (better option); add herbs such as coriander and chives, and pepper to aid in digestion (optional: small amount of hard cheese)
2. One piece of low-glycemic toast (gluten-free option as well)
3. Eggs and baked beans (gluten free when possible)
4. Low-glycemic toast with avocado, tomato, and hard cheese

5. Natural plain yogurt or coconut yogurt if you don't do dairy or are trying to cut down on dairy, fresh fruit, five to six nuts
6. Coconut Yogurt

Coconut Yogurt Recipe (courtesy of nomnompaleo.com)

- 1 can or 13.5 oz. full-fat coconut milk (Organic Native Forest is great)
- 1 tbsp. Inner-Eco fermented coconut water, probiotic kefir, or 1 capsule of any probiotic to use as your starter
- A lidded glass jar big enough to hold the contents of the can of coconut
- An oven that's free for up to 24 hours

DIRECTIONS

Step 1: Refrigerate Your Canned Coconut Milk (Optional)
Not the watery stuff in the carton—the full-fat stuff in the can. Native Forest is a good brand because they don't use BPA in the linings of their cans. If you want thicker yogurt, refrigerate the can (don't shake it up) for at least a few hours so that the cream rises to the top.

Then just use the cream and not the water at the bottom of the can. If you don't want to waste the water at the bottom of the can, you can always put it in a smoothie or…drink it?

I use the entire can of coconut milk—water and all—because I don't mind if my yogurt is a little thin. One might even call it runny. By the way, the amount of yogurt you get from this recipe is equal to the amount of coconut milk you use. So if you use an entire 13.5-ounce can, you'll get the whole 13.5 ounces, or about one and three-quarter cups.

Step 2: Combine Ingredients
Yes, there are only two ingredients! Place the coconut milk, or just the cream if you choose, into a sterilized glass jar with either the tablespoon of Inner-Eco or the contents of the probiotic capsule. If you're working with the probiotic capsule, just open it up and dump in the powder. Then mix it up with a plastic or metal spoon.

Step 3: Wait
Put the sealed jar of yogurt in the oven with the light on. *Do not turn the oven on.* Just close the oven door and turn on the oven light. Even in the midst of a freezing-cold winter in Colorado, the closed oven and the light generate a stable temperature of about 105–110 degree Fahrenheit, perfect conditions for the coconut milk to incubate.

You could also put it in a cooler with a heating pad in the cooler or covering it. The longer it sits, the more yogurt-y it becomes, so I leave mine in for twenty-four hours. Normally, you'd let dairy milk sit for seven hours after heating it up on the stove to get it to that 110 degree Fahrenheit, but I'm using a shortened preparation process here because we're all busy. It's not necessary to heat up either dairy milk or coconut milk before letting it incubate.

Step 4: Optional
Add in berries, nuts, seeds, cinnamon, and because of the high good fat content, even adding a *small amount* of honey occasionally is also an acceptable option.

Coconut yogurt is an excellent source of good fats, good protein, and low GI/GL carbs especially when you make it yourself. There is a significant amount of saturated fat in coconut, so many think it is unhealthy. But saturated fat, as we discussed before, has gotten a bad rap regarding its relationship to cardiovascular disease (heart health). Saturated fat especially from nonanimal products has never been shown to increase cardiovascular disease, and recent evidence shows the association to cardiovascular disease from animal-based saturated fat has come into question. So bottom line—enjoy your coconut!

7. Muesli (gluten-free option available as well) with yogurt. Buy the ingredients separately yourself and mix it together so you know there are no fillers or extra sugars and other synthetic ingredients to keep up its shelf life.
8. Low GI cereal (gluten free options available) with powdered cinnamon, add raw nuts, seeds, and sprinkle with vanilla protein powder or a protein green smoothie mixed with water and coconut milk on the side.
9. Protein smoothie: Whey, rice bran or pea protein, natural yogurt, crushed ice, coconut milk, egg (optional), banana, small amount of organic cocoa and/or powdered cinnamon. You can also add another fruit and/or nuts if desired.

EXAMPLES OF MORNING TEA OR SNACK

1. Five to six raw nuts and variety of seeds
2. Low-glycemic fruits, such as apple or pear
3. Natural yogurt and fruit or plain
4. Rice crackers (gluten free option) and avocado, tomato, cheese
5. Carrot, celery, or low GI gluten free crackers with hummus, piece of hard cheese, or low-sodium salsa
6. Bowl of freshly made organic popcorn, small protein powder with water, or small protein smoothie

EXAMPLES OF LUNCH

1. Salad: Lettuce (various types), one to three servings (servings are the size of the palm of your hand), spinach one serving, small handful of olives, two to three small cubes feta cheese, one to two slices of avocado, capsicum, carrot, chickpeas, hard-boiled eggs, other veggies, or salads with vinaigrette dressing (option: nuts or seeds, chicken, or turkey).
2. Wrap: Gluten Free corn tortilla with above ingredients
3. Leftovers from dinner: Protein and vegetables
4. Homemade (organic if possible) soup with lentils/beans, variety of vegetables. If having bread, one to two slices of low-glycemic gluten free bread. If not eating bread, add a salad with chicken.
5. Turkey, chicken, or other lean meat or egg with hummus or avocado and two to three vegetables or salads

EXAMPLES FOR AFTERNOON TEA/SNACK
See morning tea.

EXAMPLES OF DINNERS

1. Meat and three to four vegetables and/or salads. No breads.
2. Once a week—a small amount of gluten free pasta with chicken, vegetables, light white sauce or light red sauce
3. Stir fry (once a week with low GI rice), various vegetables, cruciferous vegetables lightly stir-fried are great for supporting liver to optimize good estrogen production. When having rice, use one palm-size serving. Remember, you can have stir-fries without rice. Use fresh herbs such as lemon grass, chilies to taste, turmeric, and cardamom.
4. Vegetable pizza on gluten free base (spinach and feta, rocket and parmesan cheese)

A Very Tasty and Satisfying One-Dish Meal
This classic San Francisco dinner recipe is from *The Los Angeles Times*.

- 250 g (equivalent to 1 cup) fresh spinach, chopped; Or 300 g (equivalent to 1 and 1/3 cup) frozen chopped spinach, defrosted
- 1 tbsp. olive oil (can substitute coconut oil if concerned about reheating olive oil as this could lead to trans fat)
- 1 tbsp. butter
- 500 g (2 cups) grass-fed minced beef
- 1 small onion, diced
- 1/2 tsp. dried basil, crushed
- 1/4 tsp. mint, crushed
- 1/4 tsp. dried oregano, crushed
- 1 tsp. salt
- 1/4 tsp. black pepper
- 4 eggs

If using frozen spinach, place in a strainer and drain well. Heat oil and butter in large, heavy skillet. Add minced beef and cook, stirring, until browned and crumbly. Drain. Add onion and cook until tender but not browned. Stir in drained spinach and cook until liquid in spinach has evaporated. Beat eggs, add to meat mixture and cook, stirring, until eggs are set.
  Yield: 4 servings.

DELICIOUS LEMON CHICKEN
An easy, flavorful, low-carbohydrate dish from *The Looney Spoons Cookbook*.

- 1 cup of Greek yogurt
- 1 tbsp. minced fresh dill (or 1 tsp. dried)

- 1 tsp. lemon pepper or regular pepper
- 1 tsp. lemon zest
- 4 boneless, skinless chicken breasts

Preheat oven to 220 degree Celsius (400 Fahrenheit). Combine Greek yogurt, dill, lemon pepper, and lemon zest in a small bowl. Lightly spray olive or coconut oil in medium casserole dish. Spread a quarter of the lemon-dill sauce over the bottom of pan. Arrange chicken breasts on top of sauce in a single layer. Pour remaining sauce over chicken. Spread evenly. Bake uncovered for thirty to thirty-five minutes until chicken is tender and no longer pink.

Yield: 4 servings.

Add three of your favorite vegetables and serve.

Dinners are limited only by your imagination. There are excellent cookbooks where you can find low-glycemic, gluten free recipes to give you some variety.

Follow the guidelines outlined in this book to help you create your own dishes or choose appropriate healthy recipes from your favorite cookbooks.

Here are a few other yogurt recipes:

Nut-Milk Yogurt (Cashews, Almonds, Macadamia)

Assuming there is no nut allergy in the family, you can enjoy a nut-based yogurt for good fats, proteins, and carbs. Preparation of the nuts is a bit more labor intensive.

Follow the above recipe for coconut yogurt, but instead of the coconut milk, replace the nut milk by doing the following:

1) Soak the nuts overnight (soaking is recommended to decrease the amount of phytic acid in the nuts. Note: soaking does not eliminate this acid but can decrease it. Phytic acid has been shown to decrease the absorption of minerals zinc and iron into the body from the foods that contain this acid. However

phytic acid does *not* decrease these minerals that are already in your system.)

2) Let dry at low temperatures or in a dehydrator (optional).
3) Purchase cheesecloth or nut milk bag. Yes, there is such a thing as a nut milk bag, who knew?

(Reprinted from ohsheglows.com)

Ingredients:

- 1 cup raw almonds (after soak and dehydrated if desired)
- 3.5 cups filtered water
- 2–4 pitted Medjool dates*, to taste (I used 2 large) (optional)
- 1 whole vanilla bean*, chopped (or 1/2–1 tsp. vanilla extract) (optional)
- 1/4 tsp. cinnamon (optional)
- A small pinch of fine grain sea salt, to enhance the flavor

Directions:

1 Place almonds in a bowl and cover with water. It's preferred to soak them overnight (for eight to twelve hours) in the water, but you can get away with soaking for one or two hours in a pinch.
2 Rinse and drain the almonds and place into a blender along with filtered water, pitted dates, and chopped vanilla bean.
3 Blend on highest speed for one minute or so.
4 Place a nut milk bag over a large bowl and slowly pour the almond milk mixture into the bag. Gently squeeze the bottom of the bag to release the milk. This took me about three to five minutes to get all the milk out.
5 Rinse out blender and pour the milk back in. Add the cinnamon and pinch of sea salt, and blend on low to combine.
6 Pour into a glass jar to store in the fridge for up to three to five days or use in yogurt recipe as discussed.

Notes: If your dates or vanilla bean are dry/stiff, soak in water to soften before use. You can also use another sweetener of your choice like maple syrup. Same goes for vanilla—feel free to use vanilla extract for a more subtle vanilla flavor.

EXAMPLES OF DESSERTS
Everyone loves them, and some often crave them.

My patients' biggest worry is, "I don't want to have to give up everything," when trying to have a baby.

Coffee is one point of contention (but remember I said you can have one), and how much sugar you are consuming is another.

Many say this or that treat "is my only vice" or "I don't have sugar in my diet, except for a few desserts here and there." But when I look at these people's' food diaries, the "here and there" is often every night after dinner.

This is probably the worst time to have a treat. Studies on mice have shown eating at night or outside of an eight-hour window led to gaining weight; and although there are no great studies on whether dessert after dinner is going to be detrimental to you, it is well known that keeping your blood sugar from spiking keeps inflammation down and, therefore, could help you optimize your fertility.

But the good news is you don't have to give up dessert all together.

I don't suggest that you have dessert after dinner at home. Eating excess sugar a few hours before you go to sleep contributes to severe blood sugar swings at the time of night when you most likely are least active and then less likely to put that sugar to good use.

Having nothing to eat two to three hours before bed is preferable. Leave after-dinner desserts for a very infrequent treat, only occasionally when you are out with friends and family.

Small treats throughout the week, such as chocolate or a small amount of your favorite treat, should be eaten right after a meal that contained protein or good fat. If you have to have a treat or you feel you will just end up binging later, then allow yourself to have this once or twice a week right after lunch. It is a lot easier to tell yourself to forgo the treat today because you can have it tomorrow versus being irritated that you aren't supposed to have a treat ever again. And it's even more pointless and detrimental to look at having a treat once in awhile as being naughty or bad. I am amazed at how many adults still describe their behavior this way when it comes to having a snack.

By eliminating sugar and high-glycemic index, high-glycemic load carbs, as well as sweeteners from your diet, you will have more sustained energy and less or no lulls in energy after meals. Decreasing caffeine consumption is also key to sustaining good energy levels as well as blood sugar levels. If you do have a sweet craving, have a small piece of fruit to stop the craving. Not many people binge on apples, but it will satisfy the "I have to have it now" feeling that can sometimes overtake common sense.

Herbs such as Gymnema and Cinnamon are excellent to have before meals to address sugar cravings. Chromium is an excellent supplement, as well, to help curb sweet cravings, and, like the others, it can be taken with meals. Check with your practitioner for the best doses, especially if you are on medications that impact your blood sugar.

Fast Food Options

In this day and age, convenience is king when we are busy and trying to squeeze in appointments over the lunch hour and after work. If you are not going to be able to prepare your lunches ahead of time to eat at work or on the run, if needed, stopping at fast food places that have mostly trans fat, fried foods should be avoided.

Today, there are healthier options at some restaurants and cafes where you can choose fresh veggies, salads, and for a sandwich, a wrap, or just a salad. If you are going to a cafe, ask if they make their sandwiches and wraps fresh daily or have them shipped in. Do the best you can and choose wisely when time is short to keep yourself on track in your eating plan to optimal health and fertility. Just remember, whenever you are eating out, you have much less control and much less knowledge about the ingredients in the food you are eating. For example, azodicarbonamide is an ingredient found in many commercial breads that has been identified as a carcinogen (cancer-causing ingredient), so some fast food restaurants like Subway have decided to remove it from the breads it bakes. But other ingredients that have been linked to cancer, such as potassium bromate, are still found in the breads at some fast-food restaurants.

Though eating out occasionally can be fine, eating lunch out every day or dinner out frequently increases the chances that you are exposing yourself to endocrine (hormone) disruptors along with other potentially toxic ingredients that encourage inflammation into your. eating plan without realizing it. Your best bet—prepare your own meals as much as possible.

CHAPTER 8

STEP TWO: MINIMIZE YOUR EXPOSURE TO ENDOCRINE DISRUPTORS TO MAXIMIZE YOUR FERTILITY

In mid-2000, I gave a talk to a group of men and women who, while dealing with fertility issues, had been involved in a healthy lifestyles program at a local IVF clinic. The program helped couples focus on a holistic approach to improving their fertility. During each week of the ten-week program, there was a section that involved an expert who discussed areas often considered alternative when dealing with fertility issues. An acupuncturist, exercise physiologist, psychologist, and myself as a nutritionist and expert in complementary medicine presented to the group of couples wanting to conceive.

One night, I was outlining our Five-Step Fertility Solution with the group and began to discuss step two. Research had just been released about how certain chemicals could impact fertility and should be avoided, so I was excited to get this information out to the group, hot off the press!

The material that I thought would be empowering and useful to the audience of couples trying to conceive resulted in faces of disappointment and frustration. Not expecting this response, I asked what was going on. Why all the looks of frustration?

Most eyes darted away from mine, except for one brave soul, who said, "Well, it's just another thing to feel guilty about. I am told that my eggs are too old and that I have waited too long. I am told that I shouldn't have been doing this drug protocol, but instead I should have been doing another one, and now you are telling me I have to get rid of all this other stuff because what I have been doing at home is all wrong, too. It seems like everytime I turn around, there is something else to feel guilty about."

After a few minutes, another woman who looked just as exacerbated spoke up and said, "It is just so unrealistic. You can't avoid everything in life to try to have a baby!"

OK, I understood. I really needed to take a step back and alter my approach. Instead of basing my delivery on what I assumed would make everyone feel so excited and informed, I needed to remember what they have been through. Therefore I changed the name of step two of The Five Step Fertility Solution to Minimizing Exposure to Endocrine Disruptors since this is much more realistic.

Before I present this information, I am going to give the following warning: the information you are about to read may seem difficult at first, but it is possible to follow through. These changes over time not only benefit your fertility, but your health and your family's health for the rest of your life.

Reminder : The information in this chapter is not meant to scare you, cause you more stress, or make you feel guilty about what you may have exposed yourself to in the past. As Maya Angelou once said, "When you know better, you do better," so think of it that way. Just take a bit of information and apply that for one week, then another bit for another week, and before you know it, you have made some significant changes over time.

This chapter is meant to help you educate yourself on how you can live a healthier life and optimize your fertility in the process. Use this information to move forward, not to add stress to what can already be a terribly stressful journey. Make the changes gradually over time, and in the process, you are optimizing your health and your fertility.

What Is an Endocrine Disruptor?

The word *endocrine* means relating to glands that secrete or release hormones. According to the National Institute of Environmental Health Sciences, endocrine disruptors are chemicals that may interfere with the body's endocrine system and produce adverse developmental, reproductive, neurological, and immune effects in both humans and wildlife.

Hormones are essential for maintaining life and creating life. They are the messengers the relay information to and from cells like the eggs and sperm. Every cell in the body has receptor sites on its surface for molecules including hormones to communicate and connect with. There is an attraction between the cell and its necessary hormone. The cell and the hormone have an affinity for one another. The hormone has important information and messages for that cell to continue to function the way that it should.

Imagine a speed dating scenario. You (the hormone) pass by many cells (potential dates). It isn't until you find the one who you are attracted to and who is attracted to you that you make a connection. You, the hormone, simply pass by the other people or cells. Once connected, information is exchanged and any number of reactions can happen.

Once the appropriate hormone attaches to and communicates essential messages to that particular type of cell, reactions specific to that cell take place, which are essential to that cell's function.

But one of the problems with endocrine disrupting chemicals is they can mimic hormones. Then the endocrine disruptor instead of the hormone can bind to the cell's receptor which ultimately blocks the hormones ability to help the cell function.

If enough of that endocrine disruptor is present and either sends the wrong messages or keeps the true hormone from communicating necessary information, this can affect the function and development of those cells. Remember the eggs, sperm, ovaries, semen and endometrial lining are all made up of cells

Endocrine disruptors can impact a single hormone or several. Therefore these chemicals can impact how efficiently systems in our body work, including the reproductive system.

Endocrine disruptors can also affect organs that would normally support the reproductive system, such as the thyroid, which is located in the neck.

One example is bisphenol A (BPA). Usually found in plastics like water bottles and food containers unless they are labeled BPA-free, BPA has been proven to impact fertility by binding to cells' receptor sites and interfere with the male reproductive system. Reports of feminization of male fetuses, smaller testicles, increased prostate size, and other postnatal health issues have been identified according to the Reviews of Environmental Contamination and Toxicology report from 2014.

A study from the medical journal *Fertility and Sterility* from 2014 showed that a mother's' BPA exposure was associated with increased risk of chromosomal abnormalities leading to miscarriage.

In an article from the Brazilian Society of Endocrinology and Metabolism from 2014, endocrine disrupting chemicals were associated with premature puberty, polycystic ovary syndrome, and premature ovarian failure.

The Federation of Gynecology and Obstetrics, the first global reproductive health organization to take a stand on human exposure to toxic chemicals, also chimed in. "We are drowning our world in untested and unsafe chemicals and the price we are paying in terms of reproductive health is a serious concern," said Gian Carol Di Renzo, a medical doctor and PhD.

Government bodies, such as the FDA, report that 93 percent of the chemicals added to food lack testing for their effects on reproduction, and there is no requirement to have such testing. Therefore, it is important that individuals take responsibility for their own health and fertility by avoiding chemicals as much as possible.

Toxic Exposure: Is It Really That Prevalent?

Toxic chemicals are all around us. The US President's Panel 2009 stated, "Only a few hundred of the over 80,000 chemicals used in the USA have been tested for safety."

In April, 2013, *The New York Times* reported that the Toxic Substances Control Act is outdated and hadn't been revised since its inception in the 1970s. According to that Act, chemicals do not have to be tested for safety; they also do not have to be approved. Just whose responsibility is it to make sure that the tens of thousands, if not more, of chemicals we're exposed to are safe? Well, according to this Act, nobody is. The law currently does not require chemicals to be safe; the only requirement is that the manufacturer provides the information necessary to access the safety of a chemical—if someone wanted to do so.

The Environmental Protection Agency (EPA) can test a chemical, if it chooses. However, companies are not required to present evidence to the EPA proving the chemical is safe. The EPA can review or test chemicals for safety, but if that's not done within ninety days, the manufacturer is free to market the product, regardless.

As you can see with more than eighty-five thousand chemicals (and more being created daily), we cannot help but be exposed to some toxins.

Completely avoiding toxins really is an impossible task because it would be like avoiding air. A person would have to live in some sort of bubble! But even the plastic in the bubble would have toxins! It is, however, imperative to overall health and fertility to make your best effort to minimize your exposure.

How to Minimize Exposure

Since it is impossible to completely eliminate toxins from your life, it is important to understand what you *can* do. This includes understanding where some of them come from and the simple steps you can take over time to minimize your exposure.

Harry and Janine had been through seven fresh IVF cycles. All and all they had fourteen embryo transfers. Though the response to IVF always produced an adequate number of embryos, few embryos made it to day five or blastocyst transfer, and even these embryos when transferred just did not seem to stick.

Harry was a social smoker for many years and worked for a diesel company, where his exposure to fumes was minimal but consistent for almost a decade. They came to see me and asked what they could do to get pregnant.

CIGARETTES

Harry was surprised to hear me say his "social smoking" could be causing an issue with their fertility. It is no surprise to most people that cigarettes contain carcinogens (chemicals that cause cancer) or that they cause negative effects on the respiratory and cardiovascular systems. The labels on cigarette packages caution us that cigarette smoking is hazardous to our health. However, not everyone is aware of the full effects that cigarette smoking can have on both male and female fertility.

The American Lung Association reports that there are approximately six hundred ingredients in cigarettes. These ingredients, when burned, create an astounding seven thousand chemicals, at least sixty-nine of which are poisonous or have been proven to cause cancer. Not only are cigarettes harmful to your respiratory health, but the chemicals that are absorbed from cigarettes can actually interfere with the production of hormones in the body.

The American Society for Reproductive Medicine (ASRM) states that smoking can have a negative impact on sperm quality and quantity. Cigarettes may affect sperm count, as well as the motility and the morphology of the sperm. Cigarettes are one major source of free radicals, whether you are the smoker or are exposed to passive smoke. Smoking by the male should be eliminated even if the sperm analysis says everything looks fine. The toxins can have an impact on the DNA of the sperm or the sperm's ability to contribute to the development of the embryo. Therefore, implantation failure with IVF or a natural pregnancy may not be due to issues with the lining of the uterus, but instead the developing embryo may have a chromosomal abnormality contributed to by an unhealthy sperm and or egg.

The ASRM also states that three chemicals found in cigarettes can result in a shorter life for women's eggs. These chemicals include cyanide, nicotine, and carbon monoxide, and those are just three of the seven thousand chemicals found in cigarettes. In fact, according to a 2014 update by the ASRM, women who smoke may actually experience menopause one to four years earlier than non-smoking women. Cigarette smoking by women has also been clearly associated with taking longer to become pregnant than in women who do not smoke. Cigarette smoking has been associated with poor receptivity of the uterus as well, which means it could affect the endometrial lining and the ability of a healthy embryo to implant.

Studies have also shown an increase in erectile dysfunction and pregnancy complication rates among smokers.

Is the effect on fertility significant? Yes. In both men and women, those who smoke are twice as likely to have fertility problems. And that risk climbs even higher as the number of cigarettes smoked increases.

Cigarette smoking undoubtedly also impacts IVF success. The American Society for Reproductive Medicine reports that women who smoke require more medication to stimulate the ovaries—even so, their pregnancy rates are 30 percent less than nonsmoking women who undergo IVF treatments.

The effects of exposure to chemicals in tobacco aren't limited to cigarettes, however. Smokeless tobacco and other tobacco-related products and products that contain nicotine and the many other chemicals contained in cigarettes also impact the ability to become pregnant, the ability to carry a child full term, and the health of the unborn child. Exposure to secondhand smoke carries the same risks and effects as smoking by either partner.

While cigarette smoking is hazardous to the health of both parents, the good news is that quitting smoking can improve fertility, and the longer one hasn't smoked, the lower the rate of complications.

It is undisputed that avoiding exposure to cigarette smoke and tobacco products is one way to reduce exposure to chemicals that can and do affect fertility.

Parents Smoking Could Lead To Childhood Cancer
Smoking can also impact the health of the child if the dad was the smoker. According to a study published in the *Journal of the National Cancer Institute*, if the father smokes in the preconception period, this was associated with elevated risks of childhood acute leukemia, lymphoma, brain tumors, and all childhood cancers combined.

In the next chapter on "Optimal Supplementation", free-radical damage will be discussed. For now, it is important to know that free radicals are created through normal processes of the body. However, an overabundance of free radicals due to exposures to toxins affects the health of the cells of the body. Remember, the eggs, sperm, ovaries, testes, and endometrial lining are all made up of cells. As a double effect, cigarettes not only produce free radicals, but they also deplete antioxidants (the body's defense against free radicals) from the body.

Completely eliminating smoking, either gradually, with a patch, or cold turkey, is one of the best investments in your health and the health of your family. Some patients have found *Easy Way to Quit Smoking*, a book and audio by Allen Carr, to be an excellent resource and aid in quitting. Hypnotherapy and acupuncture have also been quite helpful for some patients trying to give up.

St. John's Wort has recently been shown to be just as effective in helping individuals quit smoking as nicotine patches, and it is cheaper. St. John's Wort is contraindicated if you are taking certain medications, so see a qualified health professional to guide you as far as dosage if you want to utilize this herb to help you quit smoking.

As previously mentioned, Harry was not convinced that their problem was his cigarette smoking. After all, he said, "I do not smoke in the house or in front of my wife, so it isn't affecting her and it won't affect the baby." After explaining the possibility that the toxins he was breathing in voluntarily each day could be affecting the embryo and its development, even though his semen analysis was within normal limits, the effects of his smoking habit began to weigh on Harry's mind. He also never thought of the fact that even though he wasn't smoking in front of Janine, the cigarette smoke was on his clothes, in his hair, and on his skin, so she was susceptible to third-hand smoke in this way. Third hand smoke is considered the contamination by tobacco smoke that lingers following a cigarette, cigar or other tobacco product being put out. It has been implicated as a potential cause of cancer just like smoking and second-hand smoke. The baby would also be exposed to this tobacco residue when Harry help the baby in his arms, snuggling up to the shirt that is full of tobacco smoker residue.

When asked if she could smell the smoke on Harry's breath when he came home, her answer was, "Yes, and I won't let him kiss me until he brushes his teeth." If she can smell it, the chemicals from the smoke are getting into her system. This type of exposure, i.e. second or third hand smoke has been correlated with fertility issues and early onset of menopause.

ALCOHOL

Both Janine and Harry would stop alcohol consumption when beginning their IVF cycles, but they continued drinking alcoholic drinks each night between the cycles. They realized this routine had actually increased since starting their fertility journey, and they were using the alcohol as a stress-management technique.

Excessive alcohol consumption can deplete the body of nutrients and in some cases create excessive blood sugar swings, therefore, having an effect on the health of the developing egg and sperm. This means that a reduction or a break from having alcohol all together may be beneficial for a period of time before conception takes place to work toward optimizing the health of the follicle, egg, and endometrial lining, as well as the semen and sperm.

Sperm can take up to three months to develop, and the female's follicles, which carry the eggs as they develop, can take up to eight menstrual cycles before the follicle comes up on the ovary. Therefore, excessive alcohol consumption that causes important nutrients such as zinc to be depleted from the body more easily could impact the health of the developing follicle, egg, uterine lining, and sperm.

To prepare the body for pregnancy, it is advisable that both the female and the male decrease alcohol consumption. Some people prefer to just stop drinking altogether. A study presented at the American Society for Reproductive Medicine's 2013 annual conference refers to the impact of alcohol on fertility as "dramatic." Their research found that women who drank three small glasses of wine during one-week had a 30 percent chance of conceiving. Those who drank only one or two glasses in a one-week period had a 66 percent chance of conceiving. Among women who had undergone three unsuccessful IVF cycles, those who later abstained from all alcohol went on to achieve pregnancy 90 percent of the time. Based on these figures, it is reasonable to advise women to abstain from drinking alcohol altogether when they are trying to become pregnant.

Now, a note on how excessive alcohol consumption can impact male fertility:

The oxidation of alcohol competes with testicular production of testosterone. These mechanisms lead to a subsequent decrease in semen volume and sperm density. Another factor appears to be an elevation in estrogen caused by testosterone converting to estrogen in men through increased activity of the enzyme aromatase. An increase in converting testosterone to estrogen is not good for making sperm or for prostate health.

Social or light alcohol ingestion does not appear to interfere with semen quality. However, excessive alcohol intake does have adverse effects on male fertility by causing decreased serum testosterone concentrations.

Harry and Janine made a pact. If they were going to give IVF one more go, considering the huge financial investment they had already put in without any result, they would both address the issue of toxins that they were voluntarily putting in their system.

Harry quit smoking with the help of the book *Easy Way to Quit Smoking* by Allen Carr and decreased his alcohol consumption to four or five per week, spread throughout the week. Harry also became more aware of more effective precautions he could take at work to decrease his exposure to toxins.

Janine decided to eliminate alcohol consumption altogether, saying it was easier for her to just give it up than decreasing it through the week.

The first few months were a struggle for Harry, so he started acupuncture, as well as our herbal program, and slowly, but surely, he began to feel better.

After six months on the program, I received a wonderful call from Harry, with Janine's voice in the background. "We're pregnant!" They responded with their typical amount of eggs, but more embryos made it to blastocyst (day five), and two were put back in, while the rest of the remaining blastocysts were frozen. Finally, they were seven weeks pregnant and had just had their first ultrasound to confirm that there was a heartbeat.

The general recommendation I make for alcohol consumption is zero to four drinks per week spread throughout the week. Making sure there is at least two to three alcohol-free days per week. And if the person chooses to drink, I recommend an organic wine, or spirit mixed with seltzer or cranberry juice, and, of course, avoid any mixers containing soda, soft drinks, and sweeteners, artificial or natural.

CAFFEINE

Excessive caffeine consumption can also be detrimental to health and fertility. Drinking two or more cups of coffee per day has been correlated with miscarriage.

Chlorogenic acid and caffeine have both individually and together been correlated with elevated homocysteine levels in the blood. Homocysteine in the follicular fluid or the semen has been correlated with less than optimal egg health, less than optimal sperm health, and miscarriage.

All men and women dealing with fertility issues should have their homocysteine tested—not just because it could be an indicator of less than optimal fertility, but also because it is an indicator for heart disease. Elevated homocysteine levels (nine or above) can usually be addressed by taking a folic acid supplement along with a B complex. Some doctors will prescribe up to 5,000 mcg of folic acid, but these high levels should be used with caution. Some research has suggested that too much folic acid in the system can be inflammatory. There should be a balance of folate with other B vitamins. Many times, adding just 500 mcg of folic acid or folate can yield a decrease in homocysteine.

There is a significant amount of misinformation about men and women who have a gene variation called MTHFR. Not long ago it was thought that if you had a variation of this gene or its enzyme, your body required a special type of folate called methylated folate. This has been shown to *not* be the case for all those who have variations of MTHFR. If you have an issue with MTHFR, please make sure you are seeing someone who not only says they are familiar with MTHFR but someone who is also familiar with a new field of science called nutrigenetics or nutrigenomics. This new field looks at many different gene variations and how they interact with each other in certain populations.

If homocysteine remains elevated after a few months on these extra supplements and the Five-Step Fertility Solution, you may need a special kind of methylated folate to bring the levels down. About 5 percent of the population require the methylated form of folate due to genetic variations.

If possible, removing caffeine from the diet is a good option, but if you absolutely love your cup of coffee, I recommend no more than one coffee a day without any sugar or sweetener. Perhaps adding cinnamon to coffee can give it a bit of extra flavor. And some people are finding that using The Bulletproof Coffee™ option may be something to consider as well. Bulletproof coffee consists of coffee with oils added and other fats like butter. Mix in a blender and serve. The oils consist of medium-chain fatty acids, which help keep blood sugar levels more balance for longer so it combats the glucose response that coffee alone and especially coffee with sweetener can cause. You can purchase the medium-chain fatty acids from the Bulletproof company, or my patients have found adding coconut oil and or one teaspoon of organic butter as well as cinnamon or vanilla creates a satisfying treat. They also report they no longer experience the significant drop in energy that they usually get a few hours after drinking coffee, which in the past had made them want another cup.

Depending on your genetic makeup, caffeine can take a very long time to be metabolized by the liver (some sources say up to seven hours for some people), so having more than one cup of Joe may contribute to inflammation in your system.

One coffee, two to three times per week (remember, no sugar or sweetener; see above for other options), is preferable so your body isn't relying on the caffeine (or sugar) hit for energy. Patients who give up coffee are oftentimes surprised at how much more energy they have when they don't drink coffee at all. I know if you rely on caffeine heavily to give you more energy you may not believe me but honestly, after a few days of headaches and sometimes fatigue energy tends to increase.

WHAT ABOUT TEA?

Black tea or black tea with milk has approximately one-third less caffeine than coffee—my recommendation is no more than one cup of black tea per day with cinnamon to help with taste and support healthy blood sugar levels.

Green tea, like black tea, is high in antioxidants (which your cells need a constant supply of to be healthy) but lower in caffeine, so one to three cups of green tea is usually fine and improve the amount of nutrients getting into your system. There is still a small amount of caffeine in green tea, so if you begin to feel too revved up on the green tea, cut back on this, as well.

Someone who drinks caffeinated beverages regularly and then gives up cold turkey can expect headaches or other withdrawal symptoms such as fatigue and or irritability for a week or so after giving up the caffeine. See your healthcare professional if the symptoms persist.

To decrease the chance of this happening, wean yourself by decreasing the amount of coffee that you have by half, until you are down to no or very few coffees per week.

Herbal teas, such as dandelion root, cinnamon, peppermint, chamomile, rooibos (pronounced roy-boss), and others are also good options for a warm drink that has positive health benefits due to antioxidant capacity and potential improvements in cellular health. You can combine the teabags for more variety. Combining apple and cinnamon, green tea and chamomile and/or peppermint, or lemon and ginger are great ways to vary the taste of your tea if you are looking for ways to increase your antioxidant content and drink more than just filtered water throughout the day.

Keep in mind, studies have shown that tea drinkers tend to be more fertile than their coffee drinking counterparts.

SOFT DRINKS AND SODAS (CAFFEINATED AND CAFFEINE-FREE)

Mark and Cindy had been trying to become pregnant for two years. When it wasn't happening, they went to their local GP, who ran the basic tests. Mark's semen analysis showed no sperm in the ejaculate. However, upon further testing, they found that he was producing sperm in the testicles, but there was apparently some damage to the vas deferens, which transports the sperm. Their only option was to take the sperm directly from the testicles and utilize IVF to fertilize the eggs produced by Cindy or use a sperm donor.

Cindy was thirty-seven with a history of having had a large fibroid removed and varying TSH levels, indicating her thyroid was sluggish. Doctors eventually diagnosed her with hypothyroidism, and she was taking a hormone called thyroxine.

Mark and Cindy had tried two IVF cycles in the United States when I met them. The doctors had told them the sperm and eggs were both of poor quality with both IVF cycles.

It was at their initial appointment that Mark revealed that he was drinking a total of ten Diet Cokes a day, and Cindy had recently given up coffee and the sugar that usually went with it, as well as soft drinks.

SOFT DRINK CONSUMPTION AND FERTILITY

As Mark's situation suggests, soft-drink consumption is still excessive. As of march 2017 Argentina tops the chart leading all other nations in soda drinking. Annually the United States has shown a drop but still US citizens on average drink an astonishing 154 litres per capita, followed by Mexico and Chile. Australia ranks twelfth with annual consumption at 82 litres per capita.

Soda or soft drinks have no nutritional value. These products are water with sugar or sweeteners, chemicals, and carbonation. These drinks, marketed as refreshing, energizing, and even diet are likely contributing to the obesity epidemic around the world. According to the Credit Suisse Research Institute, "Sugar in soft drinks is completely digested by the body without the consequential satiation of appetite that happens with solid food. In addition, sugary beverages account for over 40 percent of the added sugars we ingest."

According to the *North American Journal of Medical Sciences* there is a speculated link between the consumption of sugar-sweetened soft drinks and development of cardiovascular disease, diabetes mellitus, dental or bone problems, and obesity. At least two of those degenerative diseases are related to fertility issues, namely diabetes (or prediabetes; i.e., insulin resistance) and obesity.

Caffeinated beverages such as coffee and tea have been previously discussed. Eliminating caffeinated soft drinks would seem to be a good idea, so why not just drink energy drinks or diet soda?

Well, there are several reasons why energy drinks and diet soft drinks are not advisable, either. As discussed, there is no nutritional value at all in these products, but it is also important to consider that in mostly all these drinks, there is a chemical called bromide or bromine that is used as a common emulsifier.

Bromide or bromine has been shown to be carcinogenic (cancer causing), but it can also compete with nutrient absorption. For example, iodine is important for thyroid function. Thyroid hormones are actually composed of iodine. Iodine supports thyroid health. Both are extremely important for optimizing fertility. Diets high in products containing bromide or bromine could contribute to iodine being deficient in the system. This could, therefore, give rise to less than optimal thyroid function, which is one of the most overlooked areas regarding fertility issues.

Bromide or bromine is also commonly found in plastics and pesticides that we are all, unfortunately, exposed to in some degree. Though you cannot completely stop your exposure to bromide or bromine, you can minimize your exposure and stop drinking soda, soda pop, and soft drinks, as well as energy drinks, to help to optimize your fertility. This advice extends to flavored waters, the zero-calorie and zero-sugar drinks which is usually "code" for artificial sweetener. The term Natural on a label does not rule out chemicals in the product. The term natural is not regulated and can be used for anything.

Mark and Cindy's next IVF cycle was done after Cindy's thyroid function appeared to stabilize and Mark was off the Diet Coke for four months. They both were following the Five-Step Fertility Solution. Doctors reported his sperm showed better quality this time when they took it from the testicles. With this IVF cycle, Cindy and Mark were able to create twins, when previously they were told their embryos had little chance of surviving.

Note: Energy drinks contain large amounts of sugar and caffeine and should be avoided. Drinking filtered water preferably filtered through reverse osmosis infused with organic fruits is one of the best refreshments you can have.

PLASTICS: JUST SAY NO

Plastics have other negative effects on our health. Today we have packaged foods, bottled water, and even the refillable plastic bottles that have become the trend in our attempt to reduce waste and go green. But this increased use of plastics comes at a cost.

One example is a chemical commonly found in plastics called BPA. Since the 1960s, bisphenol A (also known as BPA), discussed earlier as an endocrine disruptor is an industrial chemical. BPA has been used in the manufacture of these plastics unless the bottles are labeled BPA-free. BPA has been proven to mimic estrogen and disrupt the hormonal balance. It is also found on receipts and in the lining of tin cans, as well as many other everyday products we are exposed to. Due to the known adverse effects of BPA, a concerted move was made to reduce the use of BPA in plastics, especially in plastics that house or encase food and drinks. The movement triggered the labeling of plastics as "BPA Free." However, a study published in *Environmental Health Perspectives* shows that the chemicals that were used to replace BPA also contain estrogen-like chemicals. Those chemicals, bisphenol S and F (often referred to as BPS and BPF), have the same ability to cause problems in reproduction, metabolism, and neurological function. It is possible that the chemicals used to replace BPA are just as bad or worse. More testing is needed. The moral of the story is don't think BPA free is enough. Minimize use of plastics and cans.

One area that we don't often think of finding BPA is on our receipts from products that we purchase. Receipts, especially, can migrate to the consumer because the chemicals can rub off onto the skin rather easily. Some suggest that, when possible, you should elect to receive an electronic receipt, rather than a printed receipt.

More frequent exposure to receipts is experienced by those who work in grocery stores and those in accounting handling these paper receipts frequently. Some health conscious grocery stores have switched to receipts made with vitamin C instead of other harmful chemicals like BPA to protect their employees, their customers and the environment.

If you don't have a grocery story that uses the BPA-free receipt paper, to avoid exposure, some people request not to be given a receipt, but when a receipt is necessary for exchange purposes or proofs of purchase, it may be beneficial to ask the cashier to drop the receipt into the bag, reducing the number of times you will be exposed to its chemicals or ask if there is an option to email the receipt. For those who are working as cashiers or in the other jobs that would require more exposure to the BPA-containing receipts, it would be a good idea to wear gloves or a glove to avoid exposure.

Here are some steps you can take to minimize your exposure to BPA, BPS, and BPF in general.

Drink from glass, ceramic, or steel	Because these products are reusable and not disposable, they are environmentally friendly without chemical additives
If you must use plastic:	- Avoid using plastic that is scratched or heavily used; - Do not wash plastic in the dishwasher; - Do not put plastic in the microwave, even if it claims to be microwave safe; - Avoid exposing plastic to extreme heat and extreme cold.
Don't buy canned foods.	- The linings of food cans contain BPA or one of its substitutes. Purchase fresh food and produce when possible to reduce exposure. Make your own soups in larger amounts and freeze the leftover soup for use later.

Plastics guide

PERSONAL-CARE PRODUCTS: WHAT GOES ON YOUR BODY, GOES IN YOUR BODY

Personal-care products are a source of chemicals that individuals voluntarily place on their body day in and day out. Few people realize that the ingredients in these products could potentially be harmful to their overall health and fertility. In an article written on legalaffairs.org, a law magazine, author Erika Kawalek discusses that in the United States, 89 percent of the 10,500 ingredients used in personal-care products have not been evaluated for safety. The 11 percent that have been tested were tested by the industry, not the government or another regulating agency. This data is corroborated by the previous information shared about the lack of testing or regulations in regard to the use of chemicals and their safety.

It is estimated by the Environmental Working Group, also known as Skin Deep, that a person uses an average of nine personal-care products on their body each day.

This would typically include the following:

- Shampoo
- Conditioner
- Soap, face or body cleanser
- Deodorant
- Toothpaste
- Mouthwash
- Shaving cream
- Hand cream
- Moisturizer, day or night cream
- Toner
- Makeup: eyeliner, mascara, lipstick, foundation
- Makeup remover
- Nail polish
- Perfume, cologne, or aftershave

Most of those products are used before you leave the house in the morning! This list doesn't include any of the products you come in contact with or are exposed to during the rest of the day. Considering that the use of personal-care products is not decreasing any time soon, it is important to investigate what exactly is going on and potentially in your body. First read the label. The first ingredient is supposed to be the most abundant ingredient in the product and it goes down from there. If you can't pronounce most or all of the ingredients and they look like scientific chemical names, chances are this is a very processed product.

For example, parabens are one of the most common ingredients considered to be potentially harmful and should be avoided. Possibly estrogenic, that is, affecting estrogen levels, parabens are often used as preservatives in personal-care products. Any derivative of the word paraben with the prefixes methyl-, ethyl-, butyl-, or propyl- should be avoided.

Here is a list of other common chemicals to look for on labels and avoid:

- Diethanolamine (DEA), potential hormone disrupter
- Triethanolamine (TEA), potential hormone disrupter
- Monoethanolamine (MEA), potential hormone disrupter
- DMDM Hydantoin, preservatives that release formaldehyde
- Diazolidinyl urea, preservatives that release formaldehyde
- Imidazolidinyl urea, preservatives that release formaldehyde
- Lanolin, if not in a certified organic product, could potentially have been exposed to insecticides from the chemicals that sheep are dipped in. Lanolin comes from sheep wool.
- Lead and heavy metals found in hair dyes
- Nonylphenols, another estrogen-like chemical being phased out of some products due to safety concerns
- Polyethylene Glycol (PEG), used in cleaning products and personal-care products

- Propylene Glycol, may be a neurotoxin (negative effect on the nervous system)

Preservatives that could potentially cause skin sensitivity, irritation:

- Benzalkonium chloride
- Cetrimonium bromide/bromine
- Quaternium-15
- Quaternium 1-29

Skin irritant and can react with other chemicals to potentially be cancer causing:

- Sodium lauryl sulfate
- Sodium laureth sulfate
- Cocamide
- Talc: Natural occurring mineral, but when inhaled can be cancer causing. Avoid using powders containing talc anywhere on the body but especially in the genital area as this has been related to ovarian cancer.
- Triclosan: used in many antibacterial soaps and present in some toothpaste. Can contribute to antibiotic resistance and issues with the hormone system, particularly the thyroid. Has been related to birth defects and weakening of the immune system. The FDA has put out a public-service announcement that antibacterial soaps are no more effective at providing protection than regular soap and water. They may contribute to antibiotic resistance as well by killing the good bacteria found on our hands as well as the bad bacteria. Our skin is an organ system and needs good bacteria to be healthy just like our gut and other organ systems in our body.
- Avoid products with the word "fragrances" on the label. Fragrance could be one of thousands of different, likely synthetic, chemicals that can contribute to health issues.

A great online resource where you can investigate the ingredients in your skin care products is www.cosmeticdatabase.com. You can either enter the specific ingredients in your personal product to see its hazard rating or enter the specific products you use. This is a great resource to start understanding what you are putting on your body.

An excellent book, *The Chemical Maze*, is a great resource guide for food additives and cosmetic ingredients. A smartphone app called Chemical Maze is also available.

MINIMIZE TOXINS: PURCHASE CERTIFIED ORGANIC PRODUCTS
Whenever possible, when buying personal-care products, buy certified organic. A good reference site for Australia is www.usenature.com. This website also offers information specific to other countries, giving many choices regarding purchasing certified organic products. In the United States, the Organic Consumers Association provides a Directory of USDA (United States Department of Agriculture) Certified Organic Body Products at https://www.organicconsumers.org/old_articles/body-care/links.php. Like any personal-care product, you may have to try a few different products from different ranges to find what works best for you.

QUICK REFERENCE FOR MINIMIZING TOXINS

- Eat fresh whole foods, certified organic, if possible. A study at Rutgers University showed that some organic produce had 88 percent more nutrients than its non-organic counterpart. The US President's Cancer Panel also sent this same message. The scientists were concerned about pesticide use and rising cancer rates among all ages, including children. Their recommendation is to give preference to foods grown without pesticides, chemical fertilizers, and growth hormones—a clear message for overall health and fertility.

If you believe it is too expensive to eat everything organic, the Environmental Working Group recommends buying the following "Dirty Dozen" as certified organic whenever possible. According to the Environmental Working Group (ewg.org) the following list of fruits and vegetables are the most heavily treated with chemicals/pesticides. See EWG.org for their list of the "Clean Fifteen" as well.

Twelve Most Contaminated
Peaches
Apples
Sweet Bell Peppers
Celery
Nectarines
Strawberries
Cherries
Pears
Grapes (Imported)
Spinach
Lettuce
Potatoes

- Eat only small fish to limit your exposure to mercury. Though fish can be abundant in good fats, larger fish can also contain high levels of mercury, which has been correlated with miscarriage. Eating fish is a great way to incorporate good fats into your eating plan, but it has to be the right kind of fish to decrease your risk of exposure to mercury, other heavy metals, and toxins.
- At least one to two times per week only eat small fish, such as whiting, sardines, and other small fish while avoiding

swordfish, shark, or tuna. To receive some of the benefits of fish without the mercury, consider taking fish oil tablets and *make sure* they have gone through the process to purify the fish oil and remove chemicals such as mercury. The phrase "mercury tested" does not always mean they have purified the fish oil. Most over-the-counter fish oil products do not guarantee that impurities are removed.

- Always rinse your fruits and vegetables in filtered water and vinegar before you eat them to at least attempt to minimize the toxins from pesticide and sprays, even if you bought organic because they can be exposed to chemicals while being transported to their final destination.
- Stay away from tinned or canned foods since BPA and other chemicals are in the lining of the cans. These chemicals and metals have the potential to seep into the foods stored in the cans.

Choices That May Not be So Obvious

- Choose the least toxic household cleaners possible. Environmentally green products are becoming more popular. You will be amazed how well vinegar and baking soda can work. See the website http://www.apple-cider-vinegar-benefits.com/cleaningwith-vinegar.html, which contains several cleaning tips with these two common household products. Other nontoxic products (used separately or combined with other natural products) that can be effectively used in cleaning include lemon juice, hydrogen peroxide, and even olive oil. For fast and easy reference, refer to the next chart to make your own household cleaners out of safe, environmentally friendly products. This information is important to improve your fertility but will be equally important when there are children in the home and when a woman is pregnant.

Product	Ingredients
Glass, window, mirror cleaner	• 2 cups water • 1/2 cup white or cider vinegar • 1/4 cup rubbing alcohol (70% concentration) Put in spray bottle and spray solution onto soft rag, not directly on surface to be cleaned.
Scouring/Scrubbing Powder *For tubs, sinks, and rust removal. Safe for porcelain and enamel – do not use on marble or granite.*	• Half a lemon • 1/2 cup borax laundry booster To use, dip the lemon into the borax and use the lemon as a sponge or scrubbing pad. Rinse when done.
Grease Cleaner *For ovens and grills*	• Pour 1/2 cup sudsy ammonia into one-gallon container Add water to produce one gallon of cleaner *How to use:* Dip sponge or mop in solution and wipe surface. Rinse with clear water.
All-Purpose Cleaner *Use on countertops and appliances*	1 quart warm water + 4 Tablespoons baking soda Mix ingredients, pour onto sponge or soft cloth and wipe area.
Marble and Natural Stone Cleaner *For use on countertops*	• A drop or two of mild dishwashing liquid (non-citrus-scented) • 2 cups warm water Mix ingredients. Using a sponge, wipe surface with cleaner and rinse. Always dry immediately

Recipes for homemade household cleaners

A word of caution: When mixing household products, always read the label to learn about any interactions or warnings. Never mix products that contain ammonia with products that contain bleach. For this can create extremely toxic fumes.

Your Nose Knows

- Beware of perfumes, nail polishes, and plastics as discussed due to exposure to another chemical called phthalates. A study has shown that women in the United States had increased levels of phthalates in their blood. Women who had these high levels while pregnant had sons who presented with smaller testicles and other issues with their reproductive system.
- Avoid commercial air fresheners, room deodorizers, and other chemical sprays in your home, office, and car as studies are finding that these chemicals can negatively affect your health and potentially your fertility. One solution to consider is the use essential oils with a diffuser. Great oils to start with are Lavender, Rose, Ylang, Ylang, and Frankincense. These are pleasant calming essential oils.

Skin Care, Hair Care, and Other Products

As discussed, check your skin and hair care products and avoid those with many synthetic chemicals. Look for organic or all natural skin and hair care products, especially when you have little ones. Keep in mind that "natural" doesn't mean healthy or good for you, so read your product labels.

Over-the-Counter Medications

If there is a natural alternative to treat minor symptoms, it is a better solution than buying a synthetic medication over the counter, especially if symptoms are just beginning. Even though advertisements tell you the over-the-counter medications will work for your symptoms and ailments, they may actually be impacting your fertility.

Many synthetic medications have side effects that impede digestion and gut function, decreasing the absorption of important nutrients for cellular health. Check with your naturopath or physician who is familiar with natural remedies to help you make the right choices for yourself.

PRESCRIPTION MEDICATIONS

There are some prescription medications that can impact male or female fertility. Always discuss with any doctor that prescribes medication for you that you are trying to become pregnant.

For example, there are certain antibiotics that should be avoided if a female is trying to become pregnant. Knowing antibiotic use can impact sperm count for a short period of time (two to eight weeks depending on the antibiotic and the dose as well as what diagnosis he has) is important.

Blood pressure medications such as calcium channel blockers were thought to be useful as a male contraceptive!

Other medications listed here can also impact fertility:

- Antidepressants
- Antipsychotics
- Sulfasalazine (used for Irritable Bowel Disease (IBD))
- Allopurinol (for gout)
- Non steroidal anti-inflammatory drugs (NSAIDS) (often used for arthritis or joint pain)
- Prednisolone and other steroids if taken in higher doses for longer term.
- Cyclophosphamide (used for autoimmune conditions)
- Antiepileptic drugs (used to prevent seizure in epilepsy but can be used for other medical issues as well)
- Blood pressure medications
- Chemotherapy
- Radiation

Always ask your physician *and* pharmacist if the prescription drug you are taking could impact your fertility. Follow up with your own research on the medication as well. This is the one time google.com may be helpful to bring issues with a medication to your doctor's attention or at the very least bring information you find on google.com and ask your physician to look into it more for you.

If the doctor says it won't impact your fertility, ask him or her for studies that show the medication does not impact fertility. Many drugs have not been tested to see whether they have an impact on male or female fertility.

Ask your pharmacist what fillers are contained in any prescription drugs that you may be taking. These drugs can contain gluten, soy, corn, or other fillers. If you have a sensitivity to these additives, it could be impacting your health.

Never stop taking any medications without consulting with your prescribing medical doctor.

PERSONAL HYGIENE PRODUCTS

Unfortunately, endocrine disruptors can be lurking around your normal everyday products, so it is important to educate yourself on what to look for.

➤ Purchase aluminum-free deodorants to avoid excess levels of aluminum entering your system. Often, a crystal deodorant, a natural herbal deodorant, or a combination of both can work well. Clinically, some women report eliminating breast soreness after utilizing an aluminum-free deodorant. Other ingredients found in deodorants and antiperspirants that should be avoided include the following:

➤ Parabens: A synthetic preservative that can affect hormonal balance and has been linked to birth defects.

> ➤ Propylene glycol: A softener that is petroleum based and can affect the nervous system, heart, and liver.
> ➤ Phthalates: They improve product consistency but has been linked to increased risk of birth defects, may disrupt hormone receptors, and increase cell mutation. Phthalates can also be found in some fragrances, cosmetics, and body care products.
> ➤ Triclosan: This is an ingredient added to antiperspirants and deodorants to prevent body odor. It is found in antibacterial soaps, sanitizing gels, and hand wipes. The United States Food and Drug Administration classifies triclosan as a pesticide and has recently stated that antibacterial soaps are not any more effective than soap and water. In addition, the Environmental Protection Agency has stated it is a possible carcinogen.

As discussed at the beginning of this chapter, all of this information may seem quite overwhelming, and you can feel like you are doing everything wrong. Just remember the quote at the beginning of the chapter by Maya Angelou, "When you know better, do better." Gradually decreasing your exposures over a period of time will be more effective for your health and fertility than avoiding this information because it frustrates you..

CHAPTER 9

STEP THREE: WHAT'S SUPP? STREAMLINE COSTS AND OPTIMIZE YOUR SUPPLEMENTATION PROGRAM

OPTIMAL SUPPLEMENTATION

CHRIS AND BARB came to see me after trying to become pregnant for two years. Chris's semen analysis had come back normal per the doctors, but on closer inspection, the abnormal forms were high at 95 percent. This may be normal from a doctor's point of view but remember it only represents 5 percent of men who created a viable pregnancy with their partners after twelve months of trying. Based on the clinical evidence, normal forms of 90–94 percent is where pregnancies often occurred in my clinic.

After looking at Barb's situation, she had many symptoms that indicated endometriosis: pain with intercourse, vomiting and diarrhea with her period, and excessive pain with her period and at ovulation.

Though it is very difficult to know if someone has endometriosis without actually doing a laparoscopy (minimally invasive surgery where the doctor goes through the belly button to have a look at the outside of the uterus, ovaries, bowel, bladder, etc.), Barb did have many of the symptoms. However, their situation was diagnosed as unexplained because of the fact that her menstrual cycle was regular and her hormone levels were in the normal range. After looking at the balance between estrogen and progesterone, the tests did show excessive estrogen when compared to progesterone, based on the optimal ratio I followed in my clinic. The high abnormal forms of Chris's sperm and the less than optimal hormone balance that Barb was displaying could have been contributing to the difficulty this couple was having in conceiving.

In the doctor's eyes, their situation was unexplained, so the next options their doctor would suggest was a drug like Clomid, and then if that didn't work, artificial insemination, and if that didn't work, IVF. Barb tried Clomiphene (Clomid) for three months and felt horrible. She decided she did not want any more medical intervention and wanted to recover from the physical and emotional rollercoaster she was experiencing, so she convinced a very skeptical Chris that they should first see me and try everything they could to conceive naturally.

During my first consultation with Barb and Chris, I discussed all the steps of the Five-Step Fertility Solution™ with them both. Chris works in IT, and throughout each day, he would sometimes have up to six coffees with sugar. He wasn't happy when I talked about cutting these down, eliminating the sugar, and gradually decreasing the caffeine to once a day or none if some of his symptoms persisted. After all, the doctor had told him everything was fine and put him on a prescription for Nexium due to reflux he was having. His doctor also suggested he cut down on the coffee and soda because it may help with the reflux, but what incentive did he have to cut down? The Nexium kept the reflux at bay most of the time, and supposedly his fertility wasn't the problem. But with 95 percent of his sperm registering as abnormal, even though this is within the "normal" range, he may have been contributing to the issue. In addition, Nexium is not a drug that was designed to be taken long term due it its effects on calcium absorption. Calcium is an important part the sperm and is necessary for the sperm to be able to fertilize the egg. Due to Nexium being related to decreasing Calcium absorption, in Chris' case it could have been affecting the sperm's ability to fertilize the egg and create a healthy embryo.

I saw Barb a few times, and she was really determined to have a baby naturally without any medical intervention. She didn't want any pills. She would only take folic acid because she said her diet was healthy, and she was scared to death to have the laparoscopy to investigate endometriosis.

It took three to four months before both Chris and Barb began to consider making the changes I was suggesting regarding their program. The biggest resistance came with the supplementation part of the program.

WHY DO YOU NEED SUPPLEMENTS IF YOU HAVE A HEALTHY DIET?

During each consult, we would have a similar conversation. Barb or Chris would ask, "Why do we have to take these supplements? We have a healthy diet. We came to you just to get the herbs."

I would explain once again that due to Chris's reflux, which was likely related to excessive sugar and caffeine consumption, his stomach health and subsequently digestion was not optimal. Also, the fact that he had been on a prescription drug like Nexium, which has been shown to deplete calcium from the system, also supports less than optimal nutrients in his system. Therefore, nutrients were potentially not being absorbed into his system as well as they should. His sperm, like every other cell in the body, needs a sufficient level of nutrients to function and be formed optimally. He may have been eating good foods, but the medications, the sugar, and the caffeine were likely affecting his gut health and contributing to inflammation.

.I also explained to Barb that unless she was able to eat all organic food, she was exposed to pesticides and other chemicals that could affect her digestion and hormone levels, so supplements and some botanicals (herbs) can help the liver process these chemicals or help to excrete or remove them from our system through urine and feces. In addition, due to the changes in farming practices and how they manage the soil on farms some research shows that foods may not be as nutrient rich as they used to be. A landmark study from the University of Texas looked at nutrient data from vegetables and fruit between 1950 and 1999. This data showed declines in the amount of protein, phosphorus, iron, riboflavin, and Vitamin C.

The convincing factor, however, came when I explained to them that if they didn't follow through with all the steps of the Five-Step Fertility Solution™, then honestly, they were wasting their time and money by utilizing only the herbal formulation. The herbs and other supplements would not be as effective if all the steps in the Five-Step Fertility Solution were not followed together.

Herbs certainly have nutrients and contribute to a person's nutrient status, but the potency of the nutrients isn't high enough to counteract the inflammation that was potentially being created with Chris' excessive coffee drinking and sugar consumption or the reason why Barb's body may not have been breaking down and getting rid of excess estrogen in her system which subsequently may have been contributing to endometriosis.

The main focus for the herbs in Barb's case was to optimize the balance of hormones estrogen and progesterone. Excessive estrogen in comparison to progesterone feeds the growth of cysts on the ovaries, endometriosis, fibroids and other estrogen dependent conditions. The main focus for Chris was to support and improve overall sperm count and quality. I then recommended that if they were not going to follow through with each of the five steps, that they stop the program and seek out another practitioner that was happy to just sell them herbs. I did not think I would see them again.

Barb and Chris did show up for another appointment. Chris explained that he was shocked when I recommended them to stop. He opened up to me that he really thought all I was doing was trying to get them to spend more money by getting the vitamin supplements along with the herbal formula. I explained to him that it was not about the money; it was about them getting the results they wanted. I was already working full time with patients day after day and had a waiting list of people. If money was the only thing I was concerned about, I would have just gone on giving them formula after formula because I knew they were fully prepared to keep taking the herbals alone, so it would have been easier and less stress for me to just let them take their herbs and see what happened. Based on research available from my clinic over the years, in many cases, herbs alone are not enough.

From that point on, Chris began to trust me a bit more and started to follow through with my suggestions, and I began to layer in an optimal supplementation program for them both over a few months.

ANTIOXIDANTS AND FERTILITY

Barb and Chris stuck to the full Five-Step Fertility Solution™ for a total of fourteen months. Gradually, Barb's symptoms related to possible endometriosis lessened to the point that her period no longer resulted in five painful days spent in bed. She still had some pain but she wasn't stuck in bed and was able to work through it.

The best outcome from being committed to the program by far was the creation of their son. I remember the tears in Barb's eyes and the proud look on Chris's face when they brought their son in to meet me when he was a few weeks old. Though the viable conception took a bit longer than what I normally see (average pregnancy on my program occurs six to eight months after being committed to the program) after Barb's symptoms were improved it took another four months to a pregnancy. They were on the program eighteen months before a pregnancy occurred. Barb was happy to have her little one and be pain-free for the first time in many years.

What I often see in the clinic is when a patient has endometriosis, having a laparoscopy to remove the endometriosis and following the program at the same time, often results in a pregnancy in the more common six to eight month timeframe.

ANTIOXIDANT BENEFITS

Medical journals, such as *Fertility and Sterility*, have published research showing the potential benefits of antioxidants related to pregnancy.

For example, two studies were published showing the total antioxidant capacity of the follicular fluid (the fluid inside the follicle where the egg is maturing) related to pregnancies in IVF; the higher the antioxidant capacity of the follicular fluid, the more pregnancies with IVF.

In addition, Japanese researchers have shown that when certain substances were oxidized in the follicular fluid creating free radicals, there were fewer pregnancies with IVF. However, when melatonin (a hormone and an antioxidant) was used at 3 mg daily prior to an IVF cycle, pregnancy rates doubled from 10 percent to 20 percent. They also noted that there was less oxidation, or free radical formation, in the follicular fluid after melatonin was taken. This may be due to melatonin's positive impact on sleep and or its impact as an antioxidant.

Therefore, this research shows the potential for antioxidants (first from our diet and second from a supplement program) to potentially improve pregnancy rates.

At times, patients will report that their doctors have said that there is nothing they can do about poor quality eggs or "old eggs." However, research supports that, like any other cell in the body, optimal nutrient status and less oxidation are correlated with improved egg and sperm health and subsequently pregnancies.

SUPPLEMENTS—TOO MUCH CONFUSION

For the consumer and even the practitioner, there is a tremendous amount of confusion regarding what supplements to take and when, as well as what these supplements can do for you.

Each nutrient or herb is usually discussed separately. What are the benefits of zinc, vitamin D, or selenium, for example? What does the herb Agnus Castus or Bacopa Monnieri do? Research on herbs and supplements is rarely discussed in the mainstream media unless a potential problem has been associated with the herb or nutrients. Often when this news hits the headlines, the full story is not shared and many are confused by what to do.

Another issue that creates confusion is researchers like to look at one nutrient or herb at a time to see what it does on its own. Nutrients and the molecules in botanicals (herbs) are synergistic. This means that one molecule relies on another molecule that may rely on another group of molecules to create its effect in the environment it grows in but also in our environment when ingested.

Our bodies use nutrient combinations to accomplish its many tasks. There are often a combination of nutrients that make one nutrient more absorbable. For example, calcium does not get absorbed well if Vitamin D, magnesium and boron are not present. And when adequate Vitamin K is present this nutrient helps to direct calcium into the skeleton instead of into places you don't want it like your organs and arteries. Vitamin C helps the body absorb iron and the list goes on. These are just of few of many examples of nutrients working in synergy.

Due to the difficulty related to separating fact from fiction in the marketing of supplements, it is very easy to have a cupboard full of half used bottles of nutrients or herbs. But it's more cost effective and more efficacious if you take supplements together that complement each other instead of thinking one super star nutrient will take care of all your issues. Though there are often certain nutrient deficiencies that may require you to take one specific nutrient (Vitamin D is an example), the majority of the time it would benefit you to find what areas in your system may be lacking and then find a combination of complementary nutrients and herbs that can assist you.

Another way of looking at how nutrients work is by considering this: If you took the most valuable player (MVP) of a team off one team and put him or her on another team without the supporting players who helped him or her be the best player, more than likely, the MVP alone wouldn't be as strong, Take Michael Jordan, for example, one of the most well-known athletes of all time who played for the Chicago Bulls and led them to several NBA championships. Once Jordan was transferred out of Chicago and wasn't surrounded by his supporting cast of phenomenal players, his teams didn't do as well. So when a pharmaceutical company removes the active ingredient (MVP) without all the supporting nutrients and other substances, the activity level of the active ingredient may not be as effective and therefore have less impact than the plant, or it may be even stronger and lead to serious side effects that would have not been experienced by eating the plant itself. Again, there are exceptions to this rule, but overall this is the case.

If you are not a sports lover, no worries—think of it this way. Will you on your own be able to have as big of an impact in life completely by yourself or does working with people, whether they be friends, employers, employees, or contractors you may hire to do work on your house or in your business, allow you to get better results and potentially have a greater impact? It certainly depends on who you are working with, though, as you will see, quality and choosing the right supplement is important as well.

Here are a couple of examples to illustrate the point that antioxidants and minerals need to work together. The mineral calcium alone does not get absorbed very well if vitamin D, magnesium, and boron are not present. Calcium also helps with the absorption of folic acid, as does vitamin B. Vitamin C helps the body absorb iron more effectively so without vitamin C in an iron supplement, some people will get constipated. And a team of nutrients, that is, selenium, zinc, iodine, and chromium, are important for the quality of thyroid hormones, which impact your fertility and overall health.

POTENCY MATTERS

Having several bottles of single supplements and herbs of varying potency in your cupboard is expensive and ineffective. It is better and more cost effective instead to have a broad-spectrum antioxidant and multi-mineral that contains optimal potency of each nutrient as supported by research.

Many supplements will contain only the amounts of the nutrients that are set forth by the government's Recommended Daily Allowance (RDA), which is established by the US government. In other countries such as Canada and Australia, this is commonly referred to as the Recommended Daily Intake (RDI). However, the RDA and RDI were developed for healthy people to prevent diseases related to nutritional deficiencies. Though these have been revised a few times over the years, these levels are not meant to combat chronic degenerative diseases of the western world such as Diabetes, which can impact fertility. Chronic inflammation, the basis of degenerative diseases also impacts hormone levels and how/if the nutrients get in and are used by our system.

So how do you know which supplements to buy?

Each country will have different upper level limits for supplements that are in a formulation. Generally, companies are not allowed to go over these limits due to the potential for health issues in the consumer. However, in the United States, the FDA, at the time of this writing, does not require supplements to be reviewed prior to them being sold. This is because of the generally safe status of most nutritional supplements. However, more and more unscrupulous companies are using adulterated (inferior) ingredients, minimal ingredients, or poor quality ingredients to save money and make a big profit. For those reasons, it is extremely important in the United States to know what you are purchasing. Therefore, here are guidelines to consider when searching for a good quality product.

- ✓ Broad-spectrum: This means that it covers a broad area and accounts for the known synergy of different nutrients. Instead of having twenty bottles of different nutrients, a broad-spectrum multi-vitamin will have several antioxidants and minerals together in one or two bottles. Streamlining supplements like this can save you money. More is not always better.

✓ Adequate Potency and Dosage: If you are going to spend the money on supplements to assist a healthy eating plan, it is important for each nutrient and herb to be at an effective potency based on current research. Dosage is also important. It is usually recommended to take supplements twice a day so the water soluble vitamins that are used up and excess excreted quickly are broken up and utilized more effectively by your system. Most one-a-day supplements are usually very low potency with the possible exception of one or two nutrients.

QUALITY SUPPLEMENTS SAVE YOU MONEY

Quality is just as important as potency. If you have the right amount of a nutrient and all the nutrients that are meant to work together to create a result but the quality of the supplement is not good or has not been tested, then you have no idea whether what you are taking is actually getting in.

✓ Pharmaceutical grade: A supplement is pharmaceutical grade if it undergoes testing to assure it can be absorbed in the body. Most over-the-counter supplements that you find at convenience stores do not do this testing, and the law does not require it. Therefore, purchasing your supplements from a trusted practitioner or directly from a company that makes supplements that are pharmaceutical grade will help ensure the supplements have been tested to get absorbed in a normal system. Ask if the supplements are pharmaceutical grade by contacting the company or practitioner selling to you.

✓ GMP: Along with being pharmaceutical grade, it is important to make sure the company that manufactures the supplements is monitored by regulating authorities and uses Good Manufacturing Practices in its factory. These are standards that help to ensure quality of the ingredients that are in the supplements by making sure the manufacturers are properly identifying the ingredients and combining them in an environment that significantly reduces the likelihood of contamination.

How do can you ensure that your supplements fall under the categories above? The best way is to find a trusted practitioner with years of experience and ask these questions:

- Are the supplements pharmaceutical grade?
- Does the supplement company follow the GMP guidelines?
- Is the combination of nutrients in the formulation based on scientific research?
- Does the company have any independent studies (not funded or done by them) to indicate the supplement's' potency, quality, and effectiveness?

It may be difficult to get the answers you seek from the practitioner, but in this day and age, all manufacturers are reachable via e-mail and their websites online. Do your own research and contact them. Sometimes you can rely on a Google search and reviews but also get the information directly from the company or find an experienced practitioner that you trust who has already done the groundwork or will do it for you.

How does improved quality save you money? Well, take a look at your cupboard. If you have supplement bottles that are half full, full or expired, or that you have thrown out because you didn't think they were helping, then buying better quality will save you money. If you are taking your supplements religiously but you have fifteen bottles a day that you are supposed to take, streamlining these with a better quality supplement and often more potent supplement will save you money. If you have never taken a good quality prenatal supplement but have not created a viable pregnancy and yet have spent money on doctor's appointments and treatments that have not yielded a result, then beginning a broad spectrum good quality prenatal along with our Five Step Fertility Solution may help you streamline or decrease some medical costs. If you have taken a prenatal consistently and have not created a viable pregnancy yet, then following through with a more in depth look at your hormone levels may help you see what you could be missing in your prenatal that may help you become pregnant faster.

INFLAMMATION AND FERTILITY ISSUES

As discussed previously, inflammation can be an enemy to optimizing overall health. Though sometimes temporary and short lived, inflammation is normal and sometimes beneficial. For example, when the skin is cut and the body creates inflammation around the wound as it heals, if the body has the nutrients and other elements to improve healing then this temporary inflammation helps the body heal. Inflammation in the form of a fever is present when your body protects itself against bad bacteria and viruses.

However, chronic long-term inflammation can result in excessive free-radical production potentially related to a poor eating plan, exposure to toxins, too much or too little exercise and nonexistent stress management. Chronic inflammation can wreak havoc on your overall health, hormones and fertility as well as contribute to accelerated aging.

Antioxidants and multi-minerals primarily from your diet and secondarily from a good quality supplementation program help oppose the inflammation, slow the aging process and improve hormone balance, overall health and fertility.

WHAT ARE FREE RADICALS?

Think of rowdy teenagers alone in a house, add some alcohol, and eventually given time, you will have damage and chaos. Free radicals (rowdy teenagers) can eventually contribute to the degeneration of cellular health (house) if left unopposed.

Antioxidants that oppose the free radicals decrease and slow down the damage and can, in some cases, repair the damage altogether. Therefore, think of the antioxidants as the police and the parents who come into the teenagers' party. They slow down or halt the damage, and the parents usually are left to clean up the mess. In summary, the antioxidants (parents and police) keep the free radicals (rowdy teenagers) in check and help keep cells healthy. Remember, eggs, sperm, follicles, ovaries, semen, and the endometrial lining of the uterus are all made up of cells, so they need to be protected from too much free radical damage to help create optimal cellular health.

For more information on the specific antioxidants and multi-minerals that are recommended at my clinic, please email your name, birth date, any medications that you may be taking, what supplements you are currently on and any diagnosis related to fertility that you may have been given to info@naturalfertility.com. I can then give you an idea of the potency of antioxidants and minerals for you and point you in the right direction. I am constantly evaluating supplements that are on the market, so if possible, I may be able to give you suggestions regarding supplements you can receive at wholesale prices. This won't be as individual of a plan that I would give in a one on one consultation process, but it can get you started.

The suggestions will vary depending on what country you live in due to limitations each country may set on potency or what supplements are available in that particular country.

Here is an example of a product that is pharmaceutical grade, broad spectrum, and potency and balance based on independent research:

Supplement	Potency
Vitamin A (as betacarotene)	15,000 IU
Vitamin C (as ascorbates)	1,300 mg
Vitamin D	1,800 IU
Vitamin E	400 IU
Vitamin K	60 ug (micrograms)
Thiamin	27 mg
Riboflavin	27 mg
Niacin	40 mg
Vitamin B6	32 mg
Folate*	500-600 ug
Vitamin B12	200 ug
Biotin	300 ug
Panthorthenic acid	90 mg
Inositol	150 mg
Choline	100 mg
N-Acetyl L Cysteine	100 mg
Bromelain	50 mg
Alpha Lipoic Acid	20 mg
Co enzyme Q10	12 mg
Lycopene	1,000 mg
Calcium (as calcium citrate)	270 mg
Iodine (as potassium iodide)	300 ug
Zinc (as zinc citrate)	20 mg
Copper	2 mg
Manganese	5 mg
Molybdenum (citrate form)	50 ug
Chromium	300 ug
Selenium	200 ug
Boron	3,000 ug

Examples of nutrients and their potency

*Folate or folic acid

Note: This is the basic nutrient potency recommendations for a multi-mineral and antioxidant formulation. However, each person is individual and may need additional supplementation if they are deficient in particular nutrients or based on their particular situation.

Here are some examples of particular nutrients for someone trying to conceive;

Over forty?

- Coenzyme Q 10 or Ubiquinol to increase the energy in the egg/sperm cell by supporting mitochondrial function.
- A supplement called pyrroloquinoline quinone (PQQ). PQQ in combination with Co Q 10 or Ubiquinol has been shown to increase the number of mitochondria in cells. And the more little engines (mitochondria) in a cell, the more energy it will have.

Been diagnosed with polycystic ovaries? You may require Inositol, selenium, zinc, and chromium.

Another person with a specific gene mutation called may require a particular form of folate[1].

The key point here is if you are going to a practitioner who is giving everyone the same thing, you are not receiving personalized recommendations. Keep in mind that finding these individual nuances in each person's system takes time and testing, which may or may not be covered by insurance. More detailed information about supplementation necessary for a particular fertility issue can be found by joining our membership website for those dealing with fertility issues: www.tipstogetpregnant.com. To find more information about what particular bonuses, discounts, and information you receive at tipstogetpregnant.com, please see the Access Now page on the website.

WHOLE FOOD SUPPLEMENTS VERSUS MULTI MINERAL AND ANTIOXIDANT TABLETS

There is a lot of controversy about whole-food supplements versus synthetic or isolated nutrient products on the market and which is better. One would automatically assume that a whole-food supplement would be better than a supplement that has utilized isolated nutrients to make up their formulations. However, that is not always the case. If a whole-food supplement company is not holding themselves to high standards of pharmaceutical grade testing by assuring their supplements are bioavailable (tested to make sure they can get absorbed in the gut), then the whole food supplement company can't assure its customers that what they are making is going to be absorbed in the system. Assuming it is better because it is a whole-food supplement is a common mistake. Keep in mind when you take a whole-food supplement, you aren't eating an orange or a potato. They must process and pack together these foods or the processed powders and create capsules or tablets. Filler are often added and in some cases not listed on the label, which can be true of any supplement due to lack of testing. So all the more reason to get to know the manufacturer.

The most important points here are twofold:

1) Investigate the company that is creating the supplements you are taking and make sure the company meets the standards that you are comfortable with. Contact them through their website.

2) If you don't have the time or want to take the time to investigate the company yourself, find a practitioner you can trust and ask them for this information. If they are recommending products, a good practitioner will have investigated the companies and be able to share with you why these products are superior. You should then be able to verify this information yourself.

3) Whole food supplements can be low potency. Compare the potencies of the nutrients to the ones listed earlier in this book to the potencies listed on the whole-food supplements or regular multivitamin.

Note Don't be afraid to ask questions but also don't be worried if the practitioner doesn't have *all* the answers. If you have a question about the product that your practitioner is not able to answer, if they believe in the product, they will go back to the company and find out the answer for you. Or you can contact the company and bring the information back to the practitioner. If they are reputable and confident in themselves, they will appreciate the information and be able to assess this from their scientific viewpoint to help you make the best decision about product.

At times, patients have brought me products that I was unaware of and upon further research found that they did in fact meet high standards—others not so much! But the point is, your practitioner should be open minded and educated, and the best scenario is a mutual respect between the two parties that works to find the best result for the patient.

Folic Acid or Folate The Good, Bad, and The Ugly

Medical professionals and the media devote a lot of time to educating people about the importance of taking folic acid before and during pregnancy to decrease the chance of birth defects developing in the baby, such as spina bifida, cleft palate, and anencephaly (an absence of a major part of the brain). However, receiving too much folic acid also could result in complications with one's health, outside of pregnancy. Too much folic acid via supplements can mask the symptoms of vitamin B12 deficiency and harm the immune system. It should also be noted that folic acid works with Vitamin C and B12 to help the body break down and use proteins, so it is important to get enough of vitamin C and B12 when taking folic acid or folate. When in doubt, always check for interactions and recommended dosages, especially when attempting to conceive or during pregnancy, to ensure you're getting sufficient doses and the supplements that your body needs.

Also note that folic acid is the man-made form of folate. It is very absorbable for many people and has contributed to the decrease in deformities caused by a lack of folate in the mother or father prior to pregnancy and the mother during pregnancy.

Concern about this using primarily folic acid instead of folate has come up regarding folic acid's ability to be utilized by someone who has a gene variation called MTHFR. I have written about this earlier in *The Baby Maker's Guide to Getting Pregnant* in step one Optimal Eating Plan but will revisit it here.

MTHFR is a gene and an enzyme that helps regulate the methylation pathway in our bodies. The methylation pathway is essential to life, and if it is not working properly, it can significantly impact our health.

If a woman has a gene variation with MTHFR C677T, then she may have an increased risk of miscarriage potentially due to an impaired ability to absorb folic acid properly. However this is where the confusion begins. Not everyone with an MTHFR variation will have an issue, and so many are too quick to recommend a special type of folate called methylated folate. But taking this can actually make someone worse and not better if more information is not gathered.

New fields of research called nutrigenetics and nutrigenomics are shedding more light on how differences in our genetics impact how we absorb or process what we eat and new information is coming into play every day. But because the fields are in their infancy, sometimes information that is preliminary is taken as fact and can cause issues if everyone follows it.

The beauty of understanding our genetics is that each person will eventually know exactly what foods may cause issues for them and what they need to eat more of to prevent disease. We will also be able to discover what nutrients we may be deficient in and what may tend to be excessive based on our genes. But one gene variation is like a leaf on a tree; it does not represent the whole picture. Therefore a variation in the MTHFR gene or enzyme is just a snapshot of one gene, and without looking at the whole system and what other variations are present in certain populations and in the individual person, we are really only guessing about what the person really needs.

Karmen found out she had an MTHFR gene mutation after she had her first child while following the Five-Step Fertility Solution. She had some genetic testing before she starting preparing her body for another pregnancy. The tests revealed she had what is referred to as a homozygous gene variation (some call it mutation) of MTHFR C677T and a heterozygous variation of MTHFR 1298C. She saw a practitioner who said "MTHFR is my thing" because she took a class on the topic and read up on some information on the internet. Karmen was given a supplement called SAMe, which is considered a methyl donor and can assist the methylation process mentioned above in some people. Within days she felt nausea with headaches and dizziness. She stopped it immediately and went to a different practitioner who put her on 5000 mcg of methylated folate. Within a few days of taking the methylated folate, she felt anxious and could not sleep. She then came back to see me, and I gave her information about the controversy that exists over giving these supplements without further and more detailed testing.

Karmen decided to forgo the detailed testing at that point, which would have consisted of the mapping of her genome (cost 199.00 USD) and a urine test called an Organic Acids test to back up and further support the evidence found in the genome testing (cost 375–475.00USD).

We had some initial blood tests done instead to assess her hormones throughout her cycle and the nutrient status in her system. I reviewed her eating plan again since she felt she had gotten off track since finishing breastfeeding and trying to manage her life with her daughter who was nearly two years old and she followed the rest of the Five-Step Fertility Solution like she did the first time around. She was pregnant within four months.

Why did she react so poorly to having the other supplements that were supposed to help her due to the issue with MTHFR? Because even though she had these two gene variations called SNPs (single nucleotide polymorphism) the rest of her genetic makeup may have made up for the variations she did have. Too many methyl groups from a high dose of methylated folate and or SAMe, threw her body into a tailspin.

So how can you get more folate if you don't want to take a synthetic form of folic acid? Methylated folate at doses of 500 mcg may be fine for you. Some prenatal vitamins have this methylated folate in them already. But most importantly, besides having a supplement, you can get more folate from your diet.

Folate is naturally found in dark green leafy vegetables and is high in lentils and other beans such as pinto beans, garbanzo beans, and black and navy beans. I would recommend avoiding processed foods that are fortified with folic acid since the foods are processed and also you may overdo it with the folic acid you are ingesting. Too much can mask other B vitamin deficiencies and some research is pointing to the possibility of too much of folic acid contributing to inflammation

If you are not sure about whether you have issues with MTHFR or you know you have a variation with MTHFR and do not know what to do about your supplementation, it is important to see a practitioner like myself who has familiarized themselves with the up and coming fields of nutrigenetics and nutrigenomics.

Fish oil: Omega-3 and Why Is It Important?

Other nutrients that have been shown to be important for our health and fertility are omega-3 essential fatty acids, which are found in fish and fish oil supplements as EPA/DHA. They are called "essential" because our bodies can't make them so we have to get them from what we eat.

Why is omega-3 important to your fertility? Every cell in the body, including the cells of the reproductive system, have a membrane made up of lipids (fat) as well as protein. This membrane (think egg shell for the female's eggs and outer layer of the sperm) is extremely important as it allows substances to get into the cell and others to exit the cell

A 2013 study of two hundred women in the *Journal of Clinical Endocrinology and Metabolism* showed that increased essential fatty acid ratios results in increased implantation rates and pregnancy rates.

A 2012 study from the medical journal the *Aging Cell* states, "Omega-3 fatty acids may provide an effective and practical avenue for delaying ovarian aging and improving oocyte quality at advanced maternal age."

Some patients have commented that their doctor has said their eggs are too hard for the sperm to fertilize (which can be an issue related to the sperm not being strong enough to fertilize the egg). This could possibly be due to the health of the cell membrane or outside wall of the egg or the sperm. Omega-3 essential fatty acids may aid in the ability of the egg to be fertilized and may aid in the sperm's ability to fertilize the egg.

An increasing number of studies validate the importance of omega-3 essential fatty acids in women who are attempting to conceive. Research has shown that these fatty acids play an important role in fertility and women's health. Some of the benefits of omega-3 fatty acids are as follows

- In a study from *Human Reproduction*, men with the highest intakes of Omega 3s had higher sperm counts.
- A study published in the journal *Clinical Nutrition* compared men with low count, low motility, and high abnormal sperm to men with normal sperm parameters who had already had a child. The study revealed that the men with lower count, motility, and morphology had much lower concentrations of omega-3 fatty acids in the system than the men with normal sperm parameter
- More recent studies conducted by the University of Illinois in 2012 revealed the importance of DHA, an omega-3 fatty acid, in male fertility. They found that DHA affects the development of acrosome, which is a structure that helps the head of the sperm penetrate the egg and contains the DNA from the father. Without sufficient DHA, the sperm will actually stop maturing, resulting in a round head that cannot penetrate the egg, instead of the pointed, cone-shaped head that is responsible for penetration. The research showed mice that were deficient in DHA and infertile were able to become fertile when they added omega-3 fatty acid supplements to their diet

Because these essential fats profoundly affect every system in the body, they are crucial to our health and fertility.

Fish Oil: More Benefits

Fish oil has also been shown in several studies to be beneficial with optimizing moods and improving sleep. As someone who has

THE BABY MAKER'S GUIDE TO GETTING PREGNANT

experienced fertility issues, I know that the stress can be unbearable at times, so anything that is healthy and can help you keep your moods balanced while trying to conceive is worth consideration.

Both physicians and patients alike have reported the improvement in patients' moods while being on our Five-Step Fertility Solution, and fish oil likely contributes to this improvement.

Because science has revealed the importance of omega-3 essential fatty acids in male and female health, in fertility, and in preg- nancy, it should not be overlooked in our daily diets. This is especially true for those in the United States, who have been found to have diets that are low in seafood and foods that contain omega-3 fatty acids. Naturally, these fatty acids can be obtained by increasing the amount of seafood, like organic wild (not wild caught or farmed) salmon. However, the mercury in seafood can be unsafe, particularly in pregnant women. Therefore, fish oil supplements are an excellent and recommended way to make sure your body gets an adequate amount of omega-3 fatty acids.

Not all fish oil is created equal, however. There are several things you should consider when investing in fish oil

1. Avoid fish oils that are low in price where the recommended dosage is several capsules per day. You usually get what you pay for when it comes to fish oil, so quality is better than quantity.
2. Purchase the brand that removes as much of the impurities as possible, including mercury. These brands are often listed *clean or purified*. Simply saying that the fish oil is mercury tested does not mean that impurities have been removed. This means the company has not removed mercury but are selling it based on what the government deems safe. However,

when trying to get pregnant, it is important to avoid mercury as much as possible. A study from the

3. The *International Journal of Obstetrics and Gynecology* compared mercury blood levels of fertile and infertile couples in Hong Kong. Blood levels of mercury were higher in those who were deemed infertile. Elevated levels of mercury in the blood have also been associated with miscarriage.

4. Avoid fish oil in clear glass since exposure to light can spoil the oils and make them rancid or rotten.

5. Choose highly-concentrated fish oils where the minimum dose is two to three capsules per day; 3,000 mg is the most common recommendation. But the concentration of the EPA and DHA is most important. EPA concentration should be a minimum of 300 mg and DHA a minimum of 200 mg in each capsule.

The cheaper brands of fish oil, you may be taking 2000–3000 mg of fish oil, but if you look at the potency of EPA/DHA, you would need to take six to nine capsules a day to take the potency necessary to support optimal health and fertility.

Note: Some people complain of burping up fish oils after taking them, and no one wants the taste of fish in their mouth all day. For most, if it is a high quality fish oil, after taking the fish oil for a week or two the burping goes away. But if one to two weeks seems like too long of a time to be reminded of your fish oil throughout the day, then try this:

Keep the fish oil in the freezer. It appears that taking a frozen fish oil decreases or eliminates the burping, most likely because it slowly breaks down in the acids of the stomach. If the burping continues, you may not be breaking down good fats very well in your stomach. You may need to consider taking a digestive enzyme that contains lipase with your fish oil and with meals that contain (preferably) good fat to help your body break down and absorb good fats more efficiently. Consult your practitioner to see if digestive enzymes are appropriate for you.

PROBIOTICS, GUT FUNCTION, AND FERTILITY

The very first step of the Five-Step Fertility Solution™ discusses an optimal eating plan. This is by far the most important step toward optimizing your health. But what happens if you are eating all the right foods, but a pregnancy is still not happening?

Patients have come to me frustrated and said, "I am eating all organic, stopped all junk food, and have given up alcohol and coffee, but I am still not pregnant."

David is a good example. A personal trainer, David was fit and healthy and had an excellent eating plan. Knowing that, I was extremely surprised to see three of his semen analyses showed 95–98 percent abnormal sperm and very low motility at twenty-eight percent. This high percentage of abnormalities and fewer number of swimmers than optimal can make it very difficult to create a pregnancy, either naturally or with assisted procedures.

Because there are millions of sperm, one can expect a certain level of abnormal sperm. However, when the level exceeds 90 percent of abnormal forms (and if the count is lower than 50 million) our stats from the clinic indicate this can be an issue with becoming pregnant naturally or with assisted procedures.

When there are high levels of abnormal sperm, this basically means that the sperm cells are not forming properly. The sperm could have deformed heads or crooked tails that could impact their ability to swim to or fertilize the egg.

Quality issues could be due to increased free radicals in the system and less than optimal nutrient absorption. This less than optimal nutrient absorption would result in the cells not having the building blocks they need to be normally formed. This in turn may be due to an eating plan that is low in important nutrients or a digestive system that is not optimally absorbing nutrients from the good foods a person is eating.

One issue I did notice with David was his digestion. Despite the fact that his eating plan was well balanced and optimum, David still complained of reflux or bloating after certain foods and occasional constipation or diarrhea.

If a person's digestion is compromised, they may have the best diet, but the foods may not be broken down efficiently. Therefore, the nutrients may not be absorbed optimally.

The first step to helping David was reminding him to slow down and chew his food thoroughly. He tended to eat very quickly, which sometimes led to indigestion. Digestion of food starts in the mouth so if a person is not thoroughly chewing their food then the stomach may not be able to break down the food as it should and this can cause indigestion.

The next step for David was to begin rebuilding his gut to optimize the absorption of nutrients into his system, starting with a multi-strain probiotic. David took this before bed, two hours after eating. He could have taken it a half an hour before food as well but he found taking it before bed easier to remember. David began to notice that he had fewer symptoms related to constipation and diarrhea, and as a bonus for both him and his wife, the flatulence he was experiencing decreased significantly.

Because he was still having some reflux issues and bloating an hour or so after eating, especially when he ate gluten containing foods, the next step was to remove gluten from his diet. Thankfully, he had not been eating many gluten-containing foods as he had noticed over the years that wheat products did not agree with him, but he was eating protein bars that contained gluten (and soy), so these were removed.

After four months on the Five-Step Fertility Solution program, David's abnormal forms had dropped to 90 percent and his motility improved to 40 percent. He and his wife decided to do IVF one more time, but opted not to have ICSI done and just utilize regular fertilization with IVF.

ICSI stands for Intracytoplasmic Sperm Injection. It is a procedure where a scientist will pick out what they believe is a healthy sperm by the way it is shaped and how it swims and then inject the sperm into the egg. Research has shown that ICSI may have increased fertilization rates, but not live-baby rates despite increasing costs. It hadn't worked in the past for David and his wife.

Without utilizing ICSI, their procedure produced fewer embryos for David and his wife. Only two made it to blastocyst stage, when in the past they had four or five. At first, this frustrated them because they thought that they had a better chance of conceiving with more embryos. However, a higher number of embryos had never created a pregnancy in the past, and the doctors had said it was probably the age of his wife's eggs, despite her only being thirty-four years old. This time, however, with fewer, but apparently better quality embryos and putting one embryo back on a fresh cycle, David and his wife created a viable pregnancy and still had one frozen embryo left.

Probiotic research is booming. More and more information is being uncovered about the importance of probiotics. The microbiome of the gut is made up of thousands of different types of probiotics (bacteria), good and bad. Research completely agrees that the gut microbiome helps support immune function and is involved in autoimmune disease. Besides this, research is showing that the anxiety and depression can be improved with probiotic administration. Every feel either of those emotions while dealing with fertility issues? In addition, specifically related to fertility, though in the very early stages of research, it has been noted that estrogen metabolism is influenced by the health of the gut and the probiotics present. All of these bits and pieces of research support the use of a good multi-strain probiotic to improve overall health and fertility.

⟋

How Herbs Helped Jenny's Gut Function and Fertility

Jenny had been off the pill for two years and despite confirming ovulation and having intercourse at the right time every month, a pregnancy had not resulted. One interesting item I found in Jenny's history was that she had a long history of chronic constipation.

There were times when Jenny would not have a bowel movement for up to ten days. Feeling extremely uncomfortable during those times, she would resort to laxatives to get her bowels moving. She was reluctant to use laxatives often because she was worried her body would start relying on them, but she felt as if she didn't have any other choice.

Jenny removed gluten from her diet, had been taking probiotics, and she had her thyroid checked. Over the years, she had two colonoscopies, and no one could tell her why she was still constipated so often and had such infrequent bowel movements. It never occurred to her that this chronic constipation could be impacting her ability to conceive.

Together we decided to focus on her gut health to decrease overall inflammation. Chronic constipation can contribute to overall inflammation in the bowel, and the bowel is in very close proximity to the female reproductive system. Because Jenny was already taking probiotics and they weren't helping, I decided to begin an herbal cleanse to help support optimal bowel health. After utilizing the herbal cleanse, which contains several herbs to optimize digestion, and another herbal supplement for optimal repair of the gut after years of constipation, Jenny also added an alkalizing greens powder to her supplementation program.

After two weeks, Jenny noticed that for the first time in her life, she had regular bowel movements, was not constipated or bloated. Her skin started to clear up and looked fantastic. Her energy levels improved, and she also reported sleeping much better.

After three months on the herbal gut cleanse, Jenny was ready to begin the process to improve her health to conceive, but before she even started the herbs for fertility (the primary goal was first to address her gut health), she found out she was pregnant.

Jenny's story helped to drive home to me how important digestion, bowel function, and nutrient absorption are in decreasing inflammation in the system, optimizing hormone levels and cellular health for overall health, as well as for fertility.

HERBS TO ASSIST WITH GUT FUNCTION

Herbs, along with probiotics, can be very effective in relation to supporting optimal digestion.

Certain herbs can act as bowel reconditioners, helping to clean out the bowel and encourage regular bowel movements.

Mucilaginous herbs, such as slippery elm, marshmallow root, and Irish moss, along with yucca, can help soothe inflammation in the gut and promote movement of fecal material through the bowel.

An article in the *Journal of the National Cancer Institute* reported that alfalfa helps to bind carcinogens in the colon to speed elimination.

Passionflower and oatstraw have been correlated with relieving nervous tension, which can contribute to irritable bowel and sleeping issues.

Horsetail helps aid digestion and has an optimal level of silica to help support the health of hair, skin, and nails.

See your healthcare professional for instructions regarding the necessity and use of these types of herbals. If you are interested in the products I utilize for a gentle cleanse and optimal gut health, please contact the clinic at info@naturalfertility.com.

HERBS TO ASSIST WITH OPTIMIZING HEALTH AND FERTILITY

Most of the time in my practice, I begin with an herbal formula to optimize health and fertility. This can be in the form of an herbal tincture, which is a liquid or in the form of tablets or capsules that contain herbs. The majority of the time, I utilize the liquid tincture for two reasons:

- It is cost effective. More herbs can go into the tincture which means fewer capsules or tablets to take.
- It provides me with the ability to individualize formulation.

When utilizing the herbal tincture, I can add or remove herbs each time I see a patient. This is dependent on how the patient is progressing and what areas still appear to need support. If patients are taking tablets or capsules, it can become more difficult to make a formulation specific for a particular patient.

Herbs that are typically used for fertility are as follows:

- **Vitex agnus-castus** or chaste tree is used to help promote fertility due to its effect on progesterone levels, and recent research also shows Vitex can support estrogen levels as well. Some will suggest taking Vitex only during the luteal phase or second part of the cycle. However, due to the fact that the follicle is what helps create progesterone and I suggest that patients who need progesterone support take this throughout their cycle since the follicle is developing in the first half of the cycle.

  If a person is utilizing Vitex for more than three months and her cycle is not regulating or she is not pregnant, further tests are needed to look into why progesterone levels may not be improving on Vitex, or, if the levels have improved, what else may be contributing the absence of a viable pregnancy. Both male and female factors need to be investigated fully.

- **Dong quai** (Angelica sinensis) has traditionally been used as a uterine tonic—an herb that supports the health of the uterus. There has been much controversy about whether or not dong quai is estrogenic, meaning that it could raise estrogen levels. However, research from several studies related to dong quai shows no effect on estrogen levels.

  An active ingredient in dong quai called ferulic acid has been shown to improve sperm quality. Therefore, dong quai can be used to support male fertility as well.

- **False unicorn root** (Chamaelirium luteum) has been a commonly used herb for fertility. In recent years, it has become endangered, and, therefore, much more expensive, and good quality is increasingly harder to find. Traditionally utilized for female fertility and optimizing both the follicular and luteal phases, false unicorn has typically been used with other herbs, such as wild yam.
- **Wild yam** (Dioscorea villosa) was thought to support progesterone, but no studies have shown this herb to have a direct impact on progesterone. Its use in creams to support the luteal phase of the cycle and its oral use have been clinically shown to improve the balance between estrogen and progesterone in some patients.
- **Shatavari**, otherwise known as asparagus root, is often used as a substitute for false unicorn. It can potentially support estrogen balance and is commonly used to optimize libido in women. In India, shatavari is a very important herb used to support fertility in women.

- **Tribulus leaf** (Tribulus terrestris) can be used to optimize both male and female fertility. Tribulus has been shown to have a balancing effect on FSH levels in women. Follicle stimulating hormone is released by the pituitary gland. In women, it is responsible for stimulating egg production. When given to women with low FSH levels, Tribulus has brought FSH up to baseline. When given to women with high FSH levels, Tribulus has been shown to be associated with bringing FSH levels down.

  In men, Tribulus is often used to optimize testosterone levels and can be a very effective herb to optimize sperm count.

  Tribulus species can vary significantly in the effect that it has on these hormone levels. It is important when utilizing Tribulus that it is confirmed that the leaf is sourced from areas such as Bulgaria and Slovakia, where the plant has been shown to have higher levels of an active ingredient called protodioscin. The varying quality of Tribulus available in the market is a good reason to go to practitioners who are familiar with where their manufacturer sources herbs such as Tribulus, helping to ensure the patient is getting the herbs with the active ingredient likely to be effective for optimizing hormone levels.

- **Damiana** (Turnera diffusa leaf) has been used traditionally as an aphrodisiac. It has also been used traditionally to address nervous tension. Sometimes when dealing with fertility issues, performance anxiety on the male can be an issue due to anxiety and putting excessive pressure on oneself to perform on command when the female is ovulating. Damiana has been helpful to some male patients in addressing performance anxiety.

Note: This is not a complete list of herbs that can be used to optimize fertility. There are many other factors to be considered when trying to understand why a couple is not conceiving or not creating a viable pregnancy. In the Bonus Info regarding "What Your Doctor Didn't Tell You About Your Fertility," I will explore these other areas and how they can be assessed and addressed by your healthcare professional.

CHROMOSOMAL ABNORMALITIES/BIRTH DEFECTS: CAN THEY BE PREVENTED?

It is now common knowledge that folic acid is an important supplement to take while trying to conceive. Research has shown that lower folic acid levels in a woman's system can be associated with babies who have spina bifida.

Spina bifida is a birth defect where the neural tube does not close, therefore, leaving the spinal cord exposed or sometimes protruding out of the area where the vertebrae are not present or split.

Research has shown that supplementing with folic acid three months prior to conceiving can help significantly reduce the development and incidence of this birth defect.

A deficiency of folic acid is also related to brain damage and cleft palate. Therefore, optimal nutrition in the diet and nutrient absorption from the gut are important for growth and development and correlated with the prevention of some birth defects.

What about chromosomal abnormalities? Can anything be done to decrease the chance of creating an embryo with chromosomal abnormalities, which is thought to be the most common cause of miscarriage?

When IVF doesn't work or when a miscarriage occurs and a chromosomal abnormality is either confirmed or suspected, most times the couple is told that it is the eggs that are the problem, but this simply is not the case. A chromosomal abnormality can just as easily be from the sperm as it could be from the egg.

Thankfully, some studies are showing that supplementation can lessen the number of sperm with chromosomal abnormalities.

In the medical journal *Human Reproduction,* it was revealed that men with higher folic acid intake had an overall lower number of chromosomal abnormalities in the sperm.

Another example is present in a study in the Oxford journal *Molecular Human Reproduction* showed that when mice were fed an antioxidant-rich diet, the oocytes (egg cells) showed less chromosomal abnormalities than the oocytes from the mice that were fed a normal diet without the antioxidant supplementation.

Therefore, when both partners follow an optimal supplementation program along with the other steps described in *Baby Maker's Guide to Getting Pregnant* as well, this could potentially decrease the chance of creating an embryo with a chromosomal abnormality where the pregnancy would not progress or may decrease the chance of creating birth defects in the developing baby.

CHAPTER 10

STEP FOUR: OPTIMAL EXERCISE PROGRAM

LET'S GET PHYSICAL! HOW EXERCISE MAY HELP OR HINDER YOUR FERTILITY

THE LAST TWO steps of the Five-Step Fertility Solution™ are the steps most often ignored. However, step four, "Let's Get Physical, How Exercise May Help or Hinder Your Fertility," is an essential part of a complete program.

In our busy society with so much technology vying for our attention, in addition to balancing our work and social life, there seems to be little time and energy left over to exercise.

Sue knew this all too well. Sue was nearly hundred pounds overweight and had tried every diet there was with very little, if any, results. Over time, she had also developed high blood pressure and was put on medication to control it.

Sue told me her number one priority in life was to have a child. After trying for four years, using Clomiphene and artificial reproductive techniques, nothing had worked. She began the distance program because she was too far to travel to my clinic, and over a period of eight months, Sue lost seventy-seven pounds and, as you will see, increased her overall health and fertility. Sue has conceived two children on the program.

How did she do it? She followed a recommended eating plan; utilized a nutritionist locally to help her stick to the plan; and for the first time in her life, Sue joined a gym and started to exercise. Joining the gym she believes is what really did the trick. She found what activities she liked to do at the gym with the help of a personal trainer, and she stuck to the program that was designed specifically for her. Sue became what she referred to as a gym junkie. She loved going to the gym. It was there that she received encouragement, and it was because of the gym that she felt she was seeing results.

Over this time, Sue's temperature charts began to change. As the weight came off, Sue began to ovulate regularly. Under her physician's supervision, she was able to come off her blood pressure medication. Once this happened, her husband decided to utilize my program as well to help with weight loss and improve his health, even though there was no known cause of fertility issues with him per the doctor.

While both partners were becoming more fit, I also noted that some cycles for Sue were a few days overdue. Her luteal phase or second half of the cycle was going on to be sixteen or seventeen days, and during those cycles, she began to feel signs of pregnancy.

It wasn't long after a few of those cycles happened that Sue and her partner created a viable pregnancy. Her total weight loss at that time was nearly eight-eight pounds.

Appropriate exercise was a key component to Sue and her partner becoming healthier and optimizing their fertility as a couple.

OBESITY, PHYSICAL ACTIVITY, AND FERTILITY

Studies have shown that obesity is one factor that contributes to irregular menstrual cycles. A study by *The Journal of Endocrinological Investigation* found that 20 percent of women of childbearing age who were diagnosed as obese have a condition called oligomenorrhea, which means light or infrequent periods. These women with oligomenorrhea had a larger waist circumference and higher body mass index and insulin levels. This is also referred to as Metabolic Syndrome. The study is one of many that confirms there is a connection between the accumulation of belly fat and irregular menstrual cycles that contribute to fertility issues.

Let's take a look at what we know about exercise and fertility: A 2013 study reported in *BioMed Central Reproductive Biology and Endocrinology* reveals that exercise can benefit fertility in both men and women. The study found that men who regularly exercise three times a week for an hour at a time had higher sperm parameters. Of significance is that the study revealed moderately active men actually had better sperm health and morphology than those who didn't exercise at all and those who exercised heavily or competitively. When a healthy diet was combined with exercise, the study found increases in sperm motility and sperm morphology.

When physical activity is combined with weight loss in overweight women, it has a protective effect on their fertility. A study reported in *Women's Health,* a medical journal in the United Kingdom revealed that obesity reduced fertilization rate and increased the risk of miscarriage, while physical activity had a positive effect on implantation and some decrease on the risk of miscarriage.

Of particular interest is the correlation between work-related activity and fertility and pregnancy. A study in the American Journal of Industrial Medicine reported physical activity is not limited to workout times, but to the level of activity we have throughout our day. When compared to those who had sedentary jobs, women whose jobs required light or medium activity had 57 to 82 percent lower miscarriage odds. Light activity in this regard includes walking or standing for a significant time, lifting ten pounds frequently, or a lesser amount very often.

EXERCISE, STRESS, AND PSYCHOLOGICAL EFFECTS

Stress is a part of our everyday life, and it is not uncommon for stress to increase when couples experience infertility. They experience an increase in anxiety and feelings of pressure including worries about diagnoses and treatments, as well as the stress of the cost of those treatments and tests. This was all in addition to worrying about not being able to become pregnant. A July, 2013, article in *BioMed Central*

Reproductive Biology and Endocrinology reports that a study of 950 men found stress has a significant impact on sperm count, motility, density, and morphology. Although, like the chicken and the egg, there is no certainty which has the greater impact—stress can impact fertility, and fertility issues can produce stress. A decrease in stress levels has been associated with an improvement in male fertility.

Though fertility issues can be stressful for both men and women, a woman's emotional stress is oftentimes more pronounced than her male counterpart. The ticking of the biological clock, the organization of blood tests, doctor appointments, temperature charting, and being surrounded by friends and family who are pregnant contribute greatly to women's psychological stress levels. Thirty percent of women who attend infertility clinics admit to being depressed or experiencing anxiety. Stressors such as these have an impact on the body, including hormonal production and balance, insulin, blood pressure, and cardiovascular health. So though I will discuss stress and how to manage it in step five, exercise is certainly an effective and unfortunately overlooked stress-management activity.

In April, 2015, the Mayo Clinic discussed how exercise reduces stress.

1. It increases the release of endorphins, which are hormones that make us feel better and experience less pain.
2. Exercise has been shown to reduce anxiety, worries, and the symptoms of depression.
3. Exercise is related to increased energy levels.
4. Exercise helps the body to function at its best. Its benefits include weight control, regulation of blood sugar (resulting in decreased inflammation), and optimizing reproductive hormone balance.

Exercise is a great, natural way to reduce stress to support optimal fertility in both partners.

Optimizing Blood Sugar Levels

Keeping your blood sugar levels in check is a huge component to decreasing inflammation in your system and subsequently decreasing physiological stress on your system as well.

Stress, as you will see in step five, "Mind/Body Connection," can impact your reproductive hormone balance, but stress on the body does not only come from emotional stress. It can also result from physiological stress due to a poor diet and lack of exercise.

Keeping blood sugar levels regulated through your eating plan is number one, but the wonderful thing about exercise is that it helps you keep your blood sugar levels regulated as well, and allows you a bit more flexibility in your eating plan because you are usually working off some of the calories that you are consuming at a much faster and more efficient rate than if you are sedentary. But let's not get crazy here. Exercise won't make up for a poor eating plan.

Exercise Improves Sleep

Lack of sleep has been associated with impaired fertility. Sleep loss can be associated with weight gain, increased stress, and decreased fertility. Prolonged sleep deprivation can also lead to increases in heart rate, blood pressure, and decreases in your brain's ability to plan, problem solve, be attentive to detail and overall poorer mental performance. Working out regularly with an appropriate exercise plan can help to improve sleep, which in turn decreases stress, optimizes weight, and improves fertility.

⌐⌐

If you are working out regularly and sleep issues are still occurring, this may be due to emotional causing adrenal stress or other sleep disturbances such as sleep apnea. Adrenal fatigue and issues with your thyroid could be affecting both your sleep and your fertility and should be addressed by your health practitioner.

⌐⌐

Sleep absolutely can affect fertility, and research supports this fact. Actually, our entire biological cycle has been based on the sun and moon (light and dark) since the beginning of our existence. Before electricity and clocks, we used the sun as a time marker. It told us when to get up, when to eat, and when to go to sleep. Our hormones reacted to the pattern of light in a very consistent, yet complex manner. It was the sleep and waking cycles impacted our hormone balance and these cycles still do today.

The medical journal *Fertility and Sterility* has explored this fact. Research shows the following:

- When you sleep (or when it gets dark), your body produces a hormone called melatonin, which is what regulates sleep and waking. Most people don't know, though, that melatonin also may have a protective effect on egg quality. When you don't sleep, your sleep cycles are disrupted, or if you sleep with the light on, your body is tricked into thinking that you're not really sleeping and the melatonin cycle is affected. A 2010 study showed the women who had higher levels of melatonin in the follicular fluid during IVF had lower levels of a poor egg quality marker 8-OHdG. The women with higher levels of melatonin from taking the prescribed 3 mg of melatonin from their physicians doubled their pregnancy rate (19 percent) versus the control group (10 percent).

  Note: People who work third shift or swing shifts have been reported to have increased fertility issues. Studies show their hormonal balances can be out of balance, their estrogen levels are decreased, and they can have more difficulty conceiving.

Sleep not only assists in keeping our hormones in check, it also affects our body's metabolism. A lack of sleep contributes to weight gain and increased inflammation, both of which affect fertility. Poor sleep is also a factor that affects marriages by way of decreased libido—being tired is one of the most common reasons for not wanting to have sex.

At a meeting of the American Society for Reproductive Medicine's research was presented that focused on sleep and IVF treatment. The research showed that change of sleep patterns can alter menstrual cycles, hormone secretions, and circadian rhythms. Studies show that too much sleep can negatively affect those undergoing IVF as much as too little sleep, suggesting that a moderate amount of sleep—at least seven or eight hours—is optimal for fertility and the regulation of hormones.

If you're having difficulty sleeping attempt the following:

1) Make sure lights from phones, computers and other devices are off in your bedroom.
2) Use a sleep mask or cover your window to keep excessive light from entering.
3) Take steps to reduce stress or anxiety that prevents you from sleeping well.

As discussed, exercise is a great way to reduce stress and expend sufficient energy to enable a deep rejuvenating sleep.

4) Avoid eating right before going to bed since this can affect the ability to go to sleep or stay asleep, so it's a good idea to eliminate snacking late in the evening and avoid spicy foods, if they tend to give you indigestion or heartburn.
5) Reducing your fluid intake before bedtime can also minimize the number of times you awaken to go to the bathroom. Remember, you're not only seeking to get enough sleep, but you're also striving for good quality sleep that gives your body the opportunity to replenish and recharge.

SHIFT WORK, SLEEP, AND FERTILITY

Studies have connected shift work and the associated change in sleep cycles with reproductive health. In 2013, the European Society of Human Reproduction and Embryology in London found that women who don't work the typical nine-to-five shift, also known as shift workers, experience more menstrual disruption and irregularities and a reduction in fertility. They also connect shift work to the increased risk of miscarriage.

According to Dr. Linden Stocker, "Anybody who works shifts has changes to their biological functioning, and it could be any one of a number of things that has an impact on [women's] ability to reproduce."

The study included 122,000 women and the results found women who worked a rotating shift had a 33 percent higher rate of menstrual disruption and an 80 percent increase in the rate of sub-fertility. Those who worked third shift, or nights, didn't experience a significant difference in menstrual issues or difficulty conceiving; however, they did carry a higher risk of miscarriage.

While the cause(s) are not yet understood, there is much we do know. First, women who work nights or irregular shifts have different lifestyles that can lend to a lack of sleep, a poor diet, inconsistent schedules, and a lack of exercise.

Keith Summa, a researcher from Northwestern University who authored a study of the fertility of mice in a study that manipulates the cycle of light and dark, called the effect on fertility "dramatic." His study published in PLoS One (Public Library of Science) showed that disruption of circadian rhythms with repeated changes in light and dark cycles decreased pregnancy outcomes.

More than fifteen million Americans work irregular or rotating shifts, and nearly one-third of companies that have extended hours of operation report an increase in female shift workers. The Five-Step Fertility Solution is extremely important for women who work these shifts to help decrease the negative effects the disturbance in the sleep wake cycle can cause.

Finding It Difficult to Fit in Exercise

1) Exercise on breaks at work. Whether it is taking a walk around the block on your brake instead of checking emails or your social media account, or climbing a few flights of stairs at work, find time to get moving and be active.
2) If you have a very active job as a shift worker, concentrate on restorative exercise such as Yoga before or after work to help create a balance.
3) Exercise before work 20-30 minutes
4) If you have a sedentary job, see if you can request or bring in a standing desk, or set your phone to notify you every 30-60 minutes. Then get up from your chair, do 10 squats or some marching in place.

Optimizing Physiology

Exercise has also been correlated with decreased levels of homocysteine in the blood. Elevated homocysteine is associated with coronary artery disease, heart attack, chronic fatigue, fibromyalgia, cognitive impairment, fertility issues, deficiency of folic acid, genetic mutations, and cervical cancer. Everyone has homocysteine in their blood. But high levels, in both women and men, have been attributed to fertility issues as well as the cardiovascular issues mentioned.

A study at the University of Warwick in England has provided the first evidence that regular exercise significantly lowers homocysteine in the blood of young, overweight women. After six months of walking briskly for twenty-four minutes a day, homocysteine was lowered by 27 percent.

Low folic acid and other B vitamins have been correlated with elevated homocysteine, or if you are taking folic acid and have high homocysteine (high homocysteine is considered to be above eight), you may need a special type of folic acid (see previous chapter on supplementation). Elevated homocysteine has been associated with poor egg health, poor sperm health, cardiovascular disease (heart attack or stroke), Alzheimer's, and other diseases.

OPTIMIZING ENDOCRINE (HORMONE) FUNCTION

Exercising regularly with an optimal program for your experience and activity level can help men and women, keep their blood sugar levels regulated which in turn decreases inflammation. As discussed previously, this can in turn help optimize their hormonal output.

A study performed in Australia and published in *Human Reproduction* reported that women who were anovulatory (did not ovulate) were put on a weekly program of exercise and dietary changes over six months with no IVF attempts. Average weight loss was twenty-two pounds, and approximately 90 percent who previously were not ovulating (sixty out of sixty-seven women) began to ovulate and spontaneously conceived and another thirty-four conceived following IVF.

Miscarriage rate dropped from 75 percent before the program to 18 percent after the program.

Improving the fitness level of men while decreasing weight could also improve male fertility by increasing hormone production of testosterone. Obesity and excess weight in men have been correlated with low sperm counts in some studies.

CAN YOU EXERCISE TOO MUCH?

The answer is yes! Excessive exercise is also an issue because too much exercise can put too much stress on your system, causing your body to go into stress mode and overwork the adrenals. Adrenal fatigue can result in excess stress hormone production, which can directly impact progesterone production. This can impact a woman's ability to ovulate regularly and create healthy egg cells.

Excessive exercise associated with low body weight and low body fat can affect the leptin/estrogen response in females and contribute to stopping ovulation as well. An extreme example of this is girls or women who are anorexic. If they are exercising excessively and this contributes to an extremely low body weight, menstrual cycles can stop altogether. Interestingly, this same phenomenon occurs in many obese sedentary women as well.

⟨⟩

If a woman is underweight but has been underweight her whole life, she will often say, "I have been underweight all my life and haven't had any problems, so why do I have to gain weight?" The general rule of thumb is if a woman is underweight, or overweight for that matter, and she hasn't created a viable pregnancy at that weight, potentially her weight could be affecting her fertility, and it should be addressed.

⟨⟩

Sometimes even when a woman is ovulating regularly, excessive stress caused by exercise or other stressors can contribute to a hormone imbalance between estrogen and progesterone, commonly known as estrogen dominance, This can impact moods, symptoms leading up the period such as sore breasts, PMS, or headaches (also around ovulation).

In men, excessive exercise contributes to adrenal stress, which can result in depletion of the hormone testosterone and contribute to the same issue that obesity and being overweight can contribute to, that is, a low sperm count.

Men who are taking steroids to become bigger with exercise can also negatively affect fertility. Taking testosterone can severely lower sperm count and in some cases cause sperm production to be shut down completely.

GUIDELINES FOR AN APPROPRIATE EXERCISE PROGRAM
So how much exercise is not too much but just right?

The answer is different for everyone, so it is important to find the level that is right for you.

Here are some guidelines:

1. Meet with a personal trainer.

    At least the first few sessions, meeting with a personal
    trainer will make sure you are exercising with good
    form to decrease the chances of being injured and be-
    gin you on a program to create the results that you
    want. But beware there are some personal trainers out
    there who think that they need push you to your abso-
    lute limits in order for you to get results. You are not
    trying out for *The Biggest Loser*, so most times over-the-
    top intense exercise is not necessary.

    You may want to interview your personal trainer
    first. Meet with them and ask them what kind of exer-
    cise program they would recommend based on the in-
    formation you give them. Let him or her know you are
    trying to conceive. Ask them if they have ever worked
    with someone trying to conceive. And obtain referenc-
    es from those people whenever possible.

2. Find a workout buddy.

    It is always easier to get up early or work out after
    work or on your lunch hour if you know there will be
    someone to encourage you to keep going, but if you
    don't have anyone that will work out with you, don't
    let that be a deterrent. You may find a good workout
    partner at the gym, on the tennis court, or in Zumba
    class that you look forward to seeing when you work
    out.

    If it works for you and your spouse or partner, be
    workout buddies with each other, using this time for

both of you to become healthier and fit while enjoying each other's company and providing each other with encouragement and support. It's a great way to keep yourselves motivated and inspired, while also knowing that you are both working to enhance fertility.

What if your partner or spouse is reluctant or doesn't want to participate in exercising with you? Don't let that stop you! Whether you're male or female, exercise is an important part of your overall health and fertility. As a bonus, know that being committed to exercising on a regular and consistent basis is one way to prepare your body for optimal fertility.

3. Aim for exercise two to three times a week for thirty to forty-five minutes.

The US Department of Health and Human Services recommends 150 minutes of exercise every week, spread out in different sessions throughout the week.

Exercising every day is often difficult to do at first, so if you start with three to four times per week, this may be more realistic to stick to in the beginning. As you begin to feel fit and have more energy, you can add other exercises, routines, and activities to make exercise a part of your everyday life.

4. Do a combination of cardio and resistance exercise.

Interval Training
Cardio: When people think of cardio exercises they often think of long sessions of aerobics or boring never-ending treadmill workouts, but these workouts are not supported by new research. Interval training is coming

out on top as a good way to get an effective cardiovascular session in.

Interval training is a great way to get the most out of the time spent exercising. You can participate in an interval training program for twenty minutes with good results. Interval training means increasing your effort for a short length of time and then slowing down your effort for the same or longer length of time. For example, you could jog for one minute and sprint for thirty seconds and repeat this over a twenty-minute period of time. You could do this on a bike, jumping rope, while swimming, or with many other forms of exercise. Another interval training program example is to warm up for three minutes on the stationary bike, then sprint on the bike for thirty seconds, and rest for ninety seconds and continue this pattern for twenty minutes. Both work well for weight loss and increasing cardiovascular fitness.

Another option for interval training was written up in the *New York Times* in 2015, citing a program called 10-20-30 training. Essentially, whether you are on a treadmill, a bike, a rowing machine or an elliptical machine, you can practice this or any interval program.

In 10-20-30 program, the beginning starts with a warm-up such as a brisk walk, easy jog, rowing or pedaling for two to three minutes. Then you begin to speed things up. The first thirty seconds you increase your output but feel relaxed, then twenty seconds of pushing yourself moderately, and ten seconds of really pushing yourself. Repeat this 30-20-10 five times then walk for two minutes. Repeat the five consecutive 30-20-10 intervals as before and cool down for one to two minutes. This should last you seventeen minutes total.

Only do this one to three times a week and don't repeat two of the interval sessions on consecutive days. Give yourself a day of resistance exercise or decreased activity on the in-between days.

Resistance exercise
Resistance exercise can be done with weights or bands or even sitting on a Fit Ball. You are getting resistance when doing weight-bearing exercises with yoga or in some cases Pilates. It is always a good idea to see a physical therapist or personal trainer for instructions on proper form when doing resistance exercise to make sure you aren't performing the exercise with the wrong form and putting yourself at risk of an injury.

Rotating the area of your body that you are working on is also a good idea to remain free of injury. You can work on legs one day and arms the next but always remember to give your muscle groups a day of rest in between resistance exercises. The only exception to this would be core exercises.

Exercises that support good abdominal and low-back strength when done with proper form can be done every day. Holding your stomach tight and your pelvis in the correct position while doing resistance exercise decreases your chance of injury.

5. Do something you like.

Work with your trainer to find some activities you enjoy. These activities will help keep you going with your exercise program. When you start working out on your own, you aren't likely to continue if you don't enjoy at least some aspect of what you are doing. If walking is your thing, then include it in your exercise routine. The same goes for swimming, tennis, aerobics, dancing, or whatever activity you enjoy.

Get creative and stay active: The gym and trainers aren't for everyone. So if cardio and resistance exercise in a gym drive you crazy or if after a while in the gym you just need a change of pace, try some of these other activities that work your cardiovascular system and involve resistance as well.

It you enjoy it, you won't think of it as exercise. Here are a few ideas:

- Hiking
- Walking out in nature
- Bike riding
- Snow or cross-country skiing
- Swimming
- Dancing
- A brisk walk
- Raking leaves, gardening, mowing grass, and such
- Golfing (walking the course)
- Yoga and stretching exercises
- Any other ways to stay active and have fun
- Cleaning even burns calories, but use non-toxic products, such as those described in step two for decrease toxic exposure.

6. Yoga and fertility.

Our next step in the program will discuss addressing stress to increase fertility and yoga could certainly be included in that chapter, but because it is also considered a form of exercise, I have included it here. But remember exercise *is* a form of stress management, so that is why discussing yoga now is the perfect transition to our next step.

Yoga is a form of exercise that may not be high intensity like an aerobics class, yet it can be as strenuous as you make it and is known to produce benefits that are conducive to optimal fertility.

Yoga exercises can be quite beneficial due to its effects on increasing blood flow, increasing flexibility and reducing tension as well as improvement in overall general well being.

Brenda Strong, a yoga instructor who specializes in yoga for fertility, created a yoga program specifically designed to help women boost fertility. The program, Strong Yoga4Fertility, focuses on stress reduction, relaxation, and nourishment of the reproductive organs.

The benefits of yoga on fertility are many according to Strong. First, yoga reduces stress, which is known to cause physical and psychological issues that can affect fertility. For centuries, yoga has been practiced to reduce anxiety and stress. In addition, yoga can have physical benefits, like muscle toning and tissue relaxation which contributes to body detoxification.

Strong's Yoga for Fertility aims to improve the circulation of blood to the lower back, hips, groin, and pelvis—all of which are areas that contribute to gynecological function. It works on the premise of relaxing the body, which calms the mind, benefits the nervous system, and reduces stress and the hormones associated with it. She even states that the practice of yoga helps women become in tune with their bodies, which can facilitate healing.

In her coaching, Strong advises that not all types of yoga and not all poses are ideal for fertility. Some are too strenuous. I agree and often advise women and men who are trying to conceive to avoid Bikram yoga, power yoga, or hot yoga for those trying to conceive because of their high temperatures and high intensity. Those who are regular participants in these practices are encouraged to decrease them to no more than once or twice a week and avoid them in the week leading up to and during ovulation for both the male and female and for one week after ovulation for the female.

Strong's Four Fields of Fertility focus on creating a connection between the mind and body with breathing and visualization techniques.

Whether sedentary or active, most men and women can practice yoga and find it to be challenging and relaxing, as well as good for the both the mind and body.

Do I Have to Stop Exercising When I Am Ovulating?

This is a common question, and the answer is no. You do not have to stop exercising leading up to ovulation or between ovulation and your next period.

Exercising regularly in a balanced program will not be a deterrent to the embryo implanting. You can continue abdominal workouts as well, whether that be Pilates and yoga, core stabilization exercises or appropriate weight training. If an embryo is going to implant, its implantation won't be impeded by these types of exercises.

Do I Have To Stop Exercising if I Am Doing IVF?

If you are having a procedure like IVF, you are usually encouraged to lay low and not do anything too strenuous leading up to egg collection and after embryo transfer. This makes most sense due to the extreme physiological stress the medications have already put on your system, and rest at this point can help the body deal with the hormon-al chaos that can ensue after IVF. Exercise can help this stress but not if it is making you more physically exhausted or if you experience discomfort. The swelling of the ovaries as egg growth is stimulated can be quite uncomfortable so some exercises may cause irritation. Certain yoga poses can help relieve stress as well. Ask an experienced yoga instructor for assistance. Keep in mind though, finding the time to just *be* after IVF or any medical procedure is probably the best medicine. Balance is key.

CHAPTER 11

STEP FIVE: MINIMIZE STRESS AND MAXIMIZE FERTILITY

"I DIDN'T BUY A TICKET FOR THIS EMOTIONAL ROLLERCOASTER" HOW STRESS IMPACTS YOUR FERTILITY AND WHAT YOU CAN DO ABOUT IT

THE UNDENIABLE MIND-BODY CONNECTION

AT TIMES, PEOPLE underestimate how the mind, that is, our thoughts, beliefs, and emotions, can impact the body. The body and mind, however, are inseparable, and strengthening this connection and as a result decreasing stress can be imperative to optimizing fertility.

University of California, Berkeley, researchers have found what they think is a critical and, until now, missing piece of the puzzle about how stress causes sexual dysfunction (think low libido in women/men and pre-ejaculation or difficulty maintaining an erection in men) contributes to fertility issues.

Scientists know that stress boosts levels of stress hormones, glucocorticoids such as cortisol, that inhibit the body's main sex hormone, gonadotropin-releasing hormone (GnRH). GnRH stimulates the secretion of luteinizing hormone (LH) and follicle stimulating hormone (FSH). When GnRH is inhibited, it can contribute to lower sperm count, ovulation disorders, and decreased sexual activity.

The new research shows that stress can increase the brain levels of a hormone called gonadotropin-inhibitory hormone (or GnIH). This hormone was discovered years ago in birds and known to be present in humans and other mammals. GnIH puts the brakes on re-production by directly inhibiting (stopping/slows down) the release of GnRH.

"We know stress affects the top-tier reproductive hormone, GnRH, but we show in fact that stress also affects another high-level hormone, GnIH, to cause reproductive dysfunction," said lead author Elizabeth Kirby, a graduate student at UC Berkeley's Helen Wills Neuroscience Institute. "This work provides a new target for researchers, a new way to think about infertility and dysfunction. The more we know, the more we can look for ways to treat it."

Heidi was a high level executive at her firm working sixty-hour weeks and always on the go. She met her husband, John, later in life. It was her first marriage and his second. He had grown kids that were already in their twenties. But Heidi did not have any children since she had not met anyone she felt she wanted to settled down and have children with. She and John found each other and were trying for six years to get pregnant. This included two IVF procedures. Heidi was now in her early forties and John was in his mid fifties.

When the couple came to me, because John had grown children he had been told his sperm was fine. When he shared with his doctor that his occupation had been a carpenter and painter for the last twenty-five years, this meant long-term exposure to toxins they decided to do a semen analysis and some blood tests. Upon examination of the semen analysis and blood tests, it was determined that he had a normal count, but he had motility issues and a thyroid problem as well. This, coupled with the fact that he had Celiac Disease, created a significant overall health issue. Finding all this out was a surprise to the couple and quite stressful.

When Heidi came to see me her symptoms indicated possible endometriosis. She had endometriosis removed in the past along with cysts on her ovaries and her symptoms gradually came back. Her stressful lifestyle with massive pressure at work often left her feeling exhausted. Did they have any room in their life for a baby?

MIND-BODY WORKSHOPS IMPROVE FERTILITY

Mainstream medical practitioner Alice Domar, PhD, paved the way toward understanding the mind-body connection and fertility issues.

According to Dr. Alice Domar's research, mind-body programs have been shown to be effective in both significantly increasing pregnancy rates, as well as reducing psychological stress.

For example, in a study conducted at the Mind Body Institute in Boston, 185 women who had been trying to conceive for one to two years were randomly placed into a ten-week mind-body group, a ten-week support group, or a control group where they were provided routine healthcare. The birth rates during the one-year follow-up period were as follows: mind-body 55 percent, support 54 percent, and control group where they were provided routine health care 20 percent. In addition, the mind-body patients reported significantly greater psychological improvements than the support or control patients.

In four published studies on several hundred women with an infertility duration of 3.5 years, 42 percent conceived within six months of completing the program, and there were significant decreases in all measured psychosocial symptoms, including depression, anxiety, and anger.

The program, Fertile Mind, Fertile Body, has shown similar results. Over a five-year period, 58 percent of those attending the weekend Fertile Mind, Fertile Body program conceived within three to six months after the program finished. Over 90 percent of the women who completed my individual sessions related to addressing stress have given birth. In order for their program to be defined as *completed*, they had to complete all tasks assigned to them and work with me one on one for a minimum of six sessions.

Heidi, who you met at the beginning of this chapter, had a feeling that stress may have been contributing to her feeling run down but until seeing me had not considered how this may be impacting her fertility. She enjoyed her job but also knew due to financial issues knew she couldn't just quit, sick back and relax. The Fertile Mind, Fertile Body program wasn't appealing to her. She just wanted to work on her hormone balance by taking the herbs and do her best to eat healthy. Heidi committed to doing meditation as much as possible to address her stress. In the meantime, John was feeling better on the thyroid medication and supplement support he had started. But stress ensued due to either too much work in his painting business or not knowing where the next contracting job was coming from.

COMMONLY OVERLOOKED

Since research is supporting the stress and fertility connection and improvements in birth rates and pregnancy rates after addressing this aspect of fertility issues, one would assume that workshops are readily available and that physicians would take the emotional aspect of fertility issues seriously. However, this area is usually grossly overlooked and mostly not considered.

Another couple, Melissa and Jeff were experiencing unexplained fertility issues for two years after experiencing a stillbirth at thirty-eight weeks. All tests were normal based on their fertility specialist. Upon further examination, I noted a slightly sluggish motility with Jeff and a slight issue with the balance between progesterone and estrogen with Melissa's case.

I had seen other couples with similar issues create a pregnancy at about the six month mark, so it was unusual to see that Melissa and Jeff were taking longer than average to become pregnant again.

When discussing their situation, both Melissa and Jeff felt as if they had dealt with the passing of their son, but the fact that doctors told them they could find nothing wrong with the baby after an autopsy and there was no explanation for the stillbirth of their son these facts still haunted them at times. Their fertility specialist suggested counseling early on after the miscarriage, and subsequently their grief counselor felt they were coping well, but the constant nagging questions in their minds and the stress of taking longer to conceive this time were wearing on them both. Neither Melissa and Jeff nor their physician thought they needed to pursue counseling again as they were functioning normally in their daily lives.

Speaking to friends and relatives didn't help much because, though they were there to listen, at times Melissa and Jeff felt as though their support system's attitude for the most part after two years was that it was really time to just let it go and get over it. (This perception is not uncommon and is experienced often by couples who have lost a child due to miscarriage or stillbirth.)

Melissa and Jeff decided to attend our Fertile Mind, Fertile Body workshop.

Note: It's not uncommon for others who have not experienced fertility issues to have difficulty understanding what a couple experiencing fertility issues is going through. Oftentimes, comments like, "What is taking you guys so long," "Just relax, and it will happen," as well as the endless array of suggestions friends and family will have can be quite wearing on a couple's resolve.

It is important to remember that anyone who has not experienced fertility issues will have no idea what you are going through, and expectations that they should will be met with disappointment. Experiencing fertility issues is a difficult and depressing journey filled with anxiety and pressure from family, friends, and a couple's own expectations.

In some studies, the stress of dealing with fertility issues and the depression that can follow has been rated the same as someone who has been diagnosed with a life-threatening condition, such as HIV/AIDS.

TEACH PEOPLE HOW TO TREAT YOU

Unless friends and family have experienced fertility issues, don't expect them to understand, although you can let them know how best to support you.

If you have a well-meaning friend who asks you if you are pregnant every time you see her and this is starting to get to you, be honest and let her know. Reassure her that you will tell her as soon as you know, but inform her that asking all the time is contributing to you feeling uncomfortable and sad as it continues to remind you it hasn't happened yet. As the famous Dr. Phil says, "Teach people how to treat you."

When a relative makes annoying comments about how long it may be taking for a baby to arrive, be honest and straightforward with them. You do not have to tell them everything you are doing, that is, medications, procedures, herbs, and so on, if you don't want to, but it is important for you or your spouse to take responsibility to let them know how their comments are affecting you. This type of communication can be done face to face, but you can also utilize e-mail or even the old fashioned way of writing a letter. Many times, writing a letter can be very therapeutic. Explain the way you are feeling and what would be best for you and your spouse in this situation. Keep it straightforward, and remember as you are writing it that they couldn't have any idea how you are feeling because they haven't experienced it.

If after communicating with your friends and family, they still continue to make comments and ignore your requests for moral support or they continue to bring up fertility issues or babies every time you speak to them, then you have a few options:

1. If this person is a family member who you cannot avoid, you may have to limit the time that you spend with them until you feel strong enough to face them and their comments. At times, one partner may be feeling stronger than the other. Have the person who is feeling more resilient at the time run interference for you or confront the family member or friend who doesn't seem to get it and ask them to stay away from the topic of children or babies for a little while.
2. Avoid putting yourself in situations where you know that person will be present until you feel more resilient and feel you can face them and their comments.

3. Work on addressing the stress of fertility issues so you have the strength to communicate with those who seem to be less than sympathetic, and let them know how you feel and what you really need from them. Strengthening your resolve works well to address those who tend to be too sympathetic as well, that is, wanting to talk about the fertility issues every time you see them when you just want to talk about and think about something other than trying to get pregnant.

When Friends Become Pregnant Before You

Sometimes you start trying to become pregnant at the same time some of your friends start trying. In the beginning you all are sharing stories of the trials and tribulations of trying to conceive and can even have a good laugh about some of the crazy things you read online. However when one by one your friends or let's say your best friend becomes pregnant before you, whether they were struggling to conceive or not, there may be some awkward moments that contribute to hard feelings and disappointment in these relationships. Well-meaning friends who become pregnant can make some of the same comments that "other people" have made to you about pregnancy. Sometimes these comments hurt just a little bit more because they are closer to you and were once your soft place to fall.

Other times friends who have struggled to become pregnant longer than usual right along with you become pregnant before you and truly understand what you are going through but when they become pregnant, in some cases your relationship becomes strained. They may not feel comfortable talking about their pregnancy in front of you because they don't want to hurt you. Or their excitement about their pregnancy gives them a bit of amnesia related to how it felt to be the one not getting pregnant. They are now part of the group you want to be part of and you can feel more isolated.

The best way, not the easiest way, to address this is by being honest with them. Let them know how you feel but also let them know what you need. If you are really happy for them that doesn't mean you still aren't sad for yourself. Tell them if you are okay talking to them about your pregnancy or not. Or let them know that you will tell them if it becomes too much. Let them know if you feel like you need to spend time away from them that you are working through your own stuff. Don't just disappear from their life without an explanation. You both will grieve the change in your relationship at that point. That is okay. It doesn't have to be forever.

In the meantime reach out for help regarding how to cope with this situation. On my membership site tipstogetpregnant.com I have a seven week audio course called "Magic". It discusses how you can get through these difficult times and let go of some of the hurt and discomfort you experience around friends and family (and strangers) who are pregnant when you are not. If you would like a free sample of this audio program please email info@naturalfertility.com and we can email that to you.

And when you get pregnant, keep these points in mind for those who are still trying. You may be the one to suggest sitting down and talking about what that person needs from you.

FERTILE MIND, FERTILE BODY

Melissa and Jeff described the Fertile Mind, Fertile Body weekend as cathartic. Up until that point, no one had talked to them about how the mind impacts the body and how stress can impact hormone levels. "I walked away from the weekend feeling lighter and more empowered about what I can do about my fertility issues than ever before. I felt that I would be okay no matter what happened."

Three months after letting go of the patterns that were only causing their lives and their bodies more stress, while negatively impacting their marriage, Melissa and Jeff became pregnant with their first of two viable pregnancies. The experience of having a stillborn baby was weighing on both of their minds prior to the workshop. If no one knew why it happened the first time, would it happen again? These were issues they were both struggling with but didn't mention to each other until the workshop. Through the exercises they learned over the weekend, Melissa and Jeff were able to let the fear of having another baby born still born go.

Heidi and John though were still plodding along with improvements in some months and symptoms returning in other months. I suggested additional testing so that Helen could see what her schedule and stress level were doing not only to her overall health, but her fertility.

Saliva and blood cortisol levels came back very low, and Heidi's estrogen levels (estradiol and estrone, two of the estrogens implicated in hormone dependent cancers) were very high.

With cortisol levels very low, this meant that her system had been dealing with significant stress for a very long period of time, and like a gas tank if it gets too low, there won't be much energy left to continue moving forward. In the case of humans, the protective effects that cortisol usually exhibits when it is a normal level become lost and even create the opposite effects when cortisol is too high for periods of time or too low.

This was a bit of a wakeup call for Heidi, and now after over a year on the program and now forty-two, going on forty-three, Heidi shifted her focus to working on her adrenals and doing what she could to balance her hormone levels by improving her stress management and taking a hard look at her career.

DECREASE STRESS, INCREASE FERTILITY

As discussed throughout this book, there are a number of ways you can decrease physiological stress and emotional stress. For example, the first three steps of the Five-Step Fertility Solution™ can address physiological stress directly:

1. Optimal Eating Plan
2. Minimizing Toxins
3. Optimal Supplementation program

These steps can reduce physiological stress on your system and result in feeling more balanced with better energy levels. What can you do to address the emotional stress that compounds the physiological stress and can impact the reproductive hormones discussed in the previous research?

Remember step four? Optimizing Your Exercise Program

Let's Get Physical!

Consider rejuvenating exercise such as yoga for female or male partners. Even if you have never done yoga before to help optimize your health and don't have a clue what to do, fear not! There is an excellent DVD called Bend, Breathe, and Conceive by Dr. Anna Davis. This can be purchased or rented through Amazon Video.

MEDITATION AND VISUALIZATION

Meditation is another option to help reduce stress and improve fertility. Meditation has been shown to improve hormone levels and overall health. Numerous studies have cited its health benefits. Meditation can be learned through many different avenues.

Workshops for meditation are becoming increasingly common and apps easily accessed on smart devices number in the thousands. So what should you start with especially if you are a beginner or have tried before but haven't been able to quiet your mind long enough to believe you are getting any benefit?

You can start with looking for a class at your local yoga studio or listen to meditation audios and videos online.

If you are interested in guided visualization instead of just quieting your mind and body in meditation and want something specific to fertility, I recommend looking into circleandbloom.com. They have programs specific to natural fertility, PCOS, and preparation for procedures such as IUI or IVF.

For some, prayer is meditative. Patients have revealed to me that for religious reasons meditation is not something they are comfortable with. I do my best to explain that meditation is not religious and not necessarily spiritual either (though it can be one or both for some). However if people are uncomfortable with these concepts, trying to find what they are comfortable with is part of my job. And regular daily prayers of gratitude and connection with God is a beautiful way to manage stress as well.

If you are looking for some apps to start with, patients of mine have recommended smart phone apps such as Simply B for $1.99 or a free app called Relax Melodies. If you find a good app or a good video channel please let me know so I can check it out and share with our membership if it fits with my program's goals.

DHEA

More and more studies are coming out supporting meditation as a way to improve overall health by supporting your adrenal hormones, specifically DHEA. DHEA is an important hormone that some doctors prescribe to work toward boosting estrogen levels in women since DHEA turns into testosterone, which is where a woman's estrogen comes from. The problem with taking DHEA is that it can cause side effects such as aggressive moods, acne on the face, neck, and shoulders, and in some cases hair loss. This is usually because either DHEA is low for a reason (adrenal stress) or DHEA isn't low at all and the hormone is just given without doing the testing to see if it necessary. When DHEA levels are normal and a woman takes DHEA, this can easily result in the side effects mentioned. If DHEA is low, the chances of those side effects are less but they can still occur if over time DHEA becomes too high since like other hormones that are taken orally, it can build up in your system if not monitored properly.

Helping your body naturally increase DHEA through stress management has never, in my experience, lead to any of the negative side effects I have seen with DHEA supplementation. Utilizing healthy stress management strategies to naturally increase DHEA levels by supporting your adrenal health has led to feeling more rested and rejuvenated.

Herbs called adaptogens along with the techniques discussed can also be beneficial for supporting healthy DHEA and cortisol levels, which in turn supports healthy reproductive hormone balance. Adaptogenic herbs such as Ashwagandha, Rhodiola, and some ginsengs can be beneficial. Caution should be taken with some adaptogenic herbs in pregnancy so this should be discussed with your doctor, herbalist or naturopath that has experience in this area.

Some tips for you to get started and get the most out of meditation:

1) Start off with meditation, quieting the mind for just a few minutes a day. If you have never meditated before and try to sit down for thirty minutes to quiet your mind, you are likely setting yourself up for failure or at least frustration. Just like working out, if you never worked out before and you think you can be an expert the first time around and workout for an hour without getting frustrating or wanting to give up, you are probably fooling yourself. Start with just two to five minutes a day, for a week whenever you think of it (unless, of course, you are driving a car or operating heavy machinery of any kind. This is not conducive to meditation). It could be on your lunch break, during a commercial, in the bathroom, or right before you fall asleep or wake up. Stop for a minute, focus on your breath, and let everything else just fall away or out of your mind.

2) Take deep breaths and close your eyes and continue to breathe deeply until you feel nice and relaxed.

3) Bring yourself into the present moment. Let deadlines and test results be a thing of the past and for just a few moments

simply be. Focus on a flower, a picture, or the blue sky. Keep breathing deeply, and for a few minutes just let time disappear.

4) Let the judgment go. If you are trying to quiet your mind and you start to think of what is on your grocery list or what is playing on Netflix that night, you haven't failed. The idea of meditation is to be nonjudgmental. This includes, first and foremost, not being judgmental toward yourself. If a thought interrupts the process of quieting your mind, smile and swipe it away like the screen on your phone. If it keeps happening, focus on your breathing and gently remind yourself that it is okay, and with more breaths just let whatever it is float away. Oftentimes in the quiet of our mind, the process of meditation will bring up some of the things we are worried or concerned about. That is okay; assure yourself you will be okay no matter what and clear your mind again.

I traveled to China on a meditation retreat where the group I was with visited monasteries and talked to monks who had been meditating two to three hours a day for decades. I asked them if anything ever disturbed their quiet mind when they meditated or how long it would be before I could quiet my mind completely for two to three hours. Every one of them responded by saying that after all these years' experience they each still have thoughts coming in while meditating, but one monk pointed out, "These thoughts are not disturbing my meditation. In fact, they are welcome visitors, but when I no longer give them attention, they float away."

5) Over time, increase the length of your meditation sessions to what works for you. How long should they be? The Dalai Lama was quoted once saying, "Everyone should meditate for thirty minutes a day. And if you don't have thirty minutes a day, because you are too busy, then you should meditate for an hour."

The amount of time you meditate at the beginning doesn't matter as long as you are taking the time to follow this practice for a period of time each day.

The point is to calm the mind through meditation or a guided visualization once a day. Find what works best for you. If you just don't have any extra time to meditate (your boss must come to the bathroom with you, I guess! ☺), here is a suggestion.

Everyone, hopefully, falls asleep at some point so when you lay down to go to sleep like you would do normally, just sit up for two to five minutes and quiet your mind before bed and work on expanding this time slightly every night. Your will sleep more soundly and more comfortably and may go a long way toward optimizing your hormone levels. Or lastly, put your earbuds in and set your device to a guided meditation and listen to that as you drift off to sleep at night.

Heidi finally decided it was her stress levels that were seriously impacting her ability to conceive, but more important, she admitted at almost forty-three now, she was also worried about her overall health going forward. She took a break from focusing on her fertility, and I would see her on a maintenance program every few months.

Well, more than a few months had passed and she e-mailed me to let me know that, lo and behold, at nearly forty-four years old, she was pregnant naturally. John's thyroid was stable, and she put her foot down at work and cut down her hours and hired some staff to help her. I was pleasantly surprised to hear that she had conceived and delivered a healthy baby girl eight years after beginning their journey. She sent me an e-mail after her daughter was born saying, "I know that the journey we started with you and the knowledge we learned about ourselves along the way got us where we are today. Perhaps had I been going down the same old path with work, who knows how I probably wouldn't be here today."

Stress management is often the most overlooked, but a significantly important step a couple can do to assist in creating a viable pregnancy.

ACUPUNCTURE AND FERTILITY

Over the years, patients have asked me what I thought of acupuncture and whether it would be valuable for them to improve their chances of conceiving. When you consider the impact that acupuncture can have on stress in the body, I wholeheartedly recommend it as a stress management technique. However, it is also important to note that one of the reasons it does help with lessening stress as a whole is because of how acupuncture can support overall health as well.

Acupuncture has been used for centuries alone or in conjunction with herbs and more recently modern medicine to treat ailments, relieve pain, and promote healing. It has also been used to treat some of the underlying causes of fertility issues.

Acupuncture has also been shown to be effective in improving the function of the ovaries in some studies. A 2012 study in the *Complementary and Alternative Medicine Journal* showed acupuncture improves blood flow which is often cited as a problem with women as they age. Improving blood flow may also, in turn, help create a rich lining in preparation for implantation and potentially improving egg health.

The effects of acupuncture can be instantaneous, but the greatest benefits are produced over time. Typically, several weeks of treatments are recommended for optimum benefit. The onset of these treatments should begin three to four months before IVF or three to six months before trying to conceive naturally. Some medical professionals encourage acupuncture for both pre- and post embryo transfers, as well as for natural conception. Acupuncture that is fertility related can continue for as long as twelve weeks after conception since there is evidence that it could help prevent miscarriage. But like everything else discussed in *the Baby Maker's Guide to Getting Pregnant,* acupuncture alone is not as effective as acupuncture while following the *Five-Step Fertility Solution.*

If you are interested in receiving acupuncture treatments to boost fertility, I strongly recommend that you ask around about who you should see. Ask friends, your doctor, and if the topic comes up about your fertility or general health with coworkers or even acquaintances, ask them, too. It is best to get a word of mouth referral, rather than just finding someone in your area from the Internet. Take independent online reviews (not just the reviews on their website) into consideration as well. If you see negative reviews check to see if they responded to them and how they responded. If they responded professionally and seemed sincere, then I wouldn't rule them out because not everyone is going to have a perfect experience. The best assessment though will come when you visit them and experience their treatment yourself.

If possible, seek out an acupuncturist who specializes in fertility issues. Though most acupuncturists would have been trained in how to treat fertility issues, those who have specialized are often more familiar with the latest research.

Does acupuncture work for all patients? Acupuncture is not a miracle cure. As mentioned, it can be an adjunct to optimizing fertility if the Five-Step Fertility Solution. On its own without any other intervention, it can result in short-term improvements, but in order for those to be long lasting and help to optimize hormone balance, it is recommended that acupuncture be consistent over three to six months and in conjunction with an overall holistic health program. Acupuncture has been shown to be beneficial for both male and female fertility.

YOUR BELIEFS ABOUT YOUR FERTILITY

Meditation, exercise, and other healthy stress relief techniques are excellent. However, because of the many beliefs in our society and the medical system that couples are running out of time, women are running out of eggs, and so on, and the physiological effects these thoughts can have on your system, it is necessary to assess your beliefs about your fertility as a couple and work toward focusing on the possibilities, instead of all the perceived limitations you have taken on since beginning the fertility journey.

Don't believe that thoughts and more so your beliefs can affect what is happening in your body? Let's look at the placebo effect for the proof.

THE PLACEBO EFFECT

The placebo effect describes the phenomena that occurs when a person is given what they <u>think</u> is a drug or procedure that can help them, but the drug or procedure is actually inert or has no known impact on the body, and the person reports improvement, even though the drug or procedure didn't have an active ingredient, or in the case of surgery, didn't repair any area of the body.

Why does this happen?

Our beliefs strongly influence our behaviors and our thoughts influence the release of hormones and other molecules in our body. Columbia University performed a study where a bogus pain-relieving cream was placed on one arm and the participants were told this cream relieves pain. On the other arm, they were told the cream had no pain relieving ability. When a hot stimulus was placed on the arm where the supposed pain-relieving cream was placed, the areas of the brain that influence the release of opiates, our bodies natural pain-relieving chemicals, were activated more so than when the stimulus was placed on the area where the participant was told the cream had no pain-relieving effect. Remember, neither of the creams had any pain relieving ingredients. What mattered most in this scenario was whether the participant <u>thought</u> the cream had the pain reliever in it or not.

Another interesting example of how strong the placebo effect can be, that is how strong our beliefs impact our body, has occurred following brain surgery. At the University of Denver, forty subjects who had Parkinson's disease, which is a degenerative disease that affects brain function resulting in balance issues, speech issues, tremors, and a whole host of other problems, underwent a surgery where they were told that the surgeon was going to transplant human neurons into their brain to help relieve symptoms of the Parkinson's Disease.

But only twenty of the participants received the actual treatment. The other twenty had a "sham surgery" which basically means they had holes drilled into their skull but no treatment was administered. A year later, whether they received the actual treatment or not, the participants reported better quality of life, but even more interesting was testing or neurological functioning was performed by medical personnel, and those who believed they had the treatment even though some of them hadn't had the actual surgery showed improvement in these objective findings as well.

For example, one woman who had the surgery but did not receive treatment, although she believed she did have the treatment, reported that she was not able to be physically active before the surgery, but a year after the surgery, she had been able to go hiking and had also been ice skating.

Does that mean that the surgery itself does nothing and is worthless? Not necessarily. What this information does mean is for many, the belief about the treatment can in some have a significant impact on the treatment results.

THE NOCEBO EFFECT

Does the opposite apply? If you don't believe a treatment will work, does it have less of a chance of working?

The answer may be yes. Enter the nocebo effect. This phenomenon occurs when a negative effect results after a non active treatment (like a sugar pill) is administered or when a participant has negative expectations about a treatment or procedure.

The nocebo effect was noted in pharmaceutical trials when patients were told about the side effects related to a medication they may or may not be taking. A portion of the participants on the sugar pill (inactive treatment) reported experiencing side effects that were expected with the active treatment. These studies were "blind," meaning the participant did not know they weren't getting the inactive treatment yet they experienced side effects of the active treatment.

Whether or not a participant ingested a pill or uses a cream on their body doesn't seem to matter. One study from the University of Mainz in Germany examined a group of 147 people who watched one of two television reports. One report was about the security of the Internet and cell phone data, and the other group watched a television report about the negative impact of the electromagnetic radio waves from every daily Wi-Fi signals.

The subjects were then exposed to fake Wi-Fi signals, which they were told were real. Fifty-four percent of the subjects reported experiencing symptoms such as agitation, anxiety, loss of concentration, or tingling in their fingers, arms, legs, and feet. Two participants left the study prematurely because their symptoms were so severe that they no longer wanted to be exposed to the assumed radiation. It was noted later that those who had preexisting diagnoses of anxiety issues responded more severely.

So your thoughts and beliefs from what you perceive and experience in life can predispose your reaction to procedures, medications, and even suggestions.

It can no longer be argued that what we believe or our thoughts don't impact the body, but instead it is well supported that the way we process those beliefs and experiences determines their individual effects on each person.

Many people say, "Come on, how can what I think and believe affect my health or physiology?" Some think this is a crazy notion. Those people in those experiments must have been a little off to begin with, right? Wrong.

I would bet you have had this experience and just never made the connection before. For example, most everyone has experienced butterflies in the stomach. Right? How did those sensations get there? What caused them?

The butterflies in the stomach feeling most likely resulted from you *thinking* about an experience you had in the past or a new experience you were going to have in the future that you were nervous or apprehensive about. Due to emotions such as fear or anxiety that you create based on your thoughts and focus about the present, past or future, you created a physiological change (cascade of stress hormones) in your system that created the physiological response, that is, butterflies in the stomach. This sensation was a result of your thoughts.

Isn't it true that men can create an erection by looking at a picture of a woman who they find attractive. This instantaneous physical response when a man is aroused is the result of what he is thinking. These thoughts resulted in the hormones cascading through his body and increasing blood flow to the penis. The hormones were produced due to the thoughts he was thinking.

Scientists have been intrigued about how some women can think themselves into having an orgasm. We all know a female organism is usually a bit more complicated than a male orgasm. According to data from brain imaging scanners, "The pleasure centers of the brain associated with orgasm light up in women who think themselves to an orgasm in exactly the same way as in women who orgasm through more conventional means," says Barry Komisaruk, who coauthored *The Science of Orgasm.*

"Some imagined erotic scenarios," Komisaruk says, "but others imagined very romantic scenes such as a lover whispering to them. Others pictured more abstract sensual experiences such as walking along a beach or imagining waves of energy moving through their body."

These are all clear examples that your thoughts and emotions can impact your hormones.

WHAT THOUGHTS OR BELIEFS ABOUT YOURSELF MAY BE IMPACTING YOUR FERTILITY?

1) I am all alone. No one else is experiencing this issue. Everyone else can get pregnant but me. Despite what you may have been led to believe, it is important to understand that what you are

experiencing is relatively common. One in six couples is experiencing fertility issues, and many need support to conceive.

2) I am infertile.

Keep in mind that if you and your partner are producing eggs (not responding to IVF drugs *does not* mean that you don't have any eggs left) and sperm, then you are not infertile! If you are 50 or over and haven't menstruated in a year, then it is highly possible you aren't producing eggs anymore, however, most reading this book would not fall into that category. Everyone else? Consider yourself fertility challenged maybe, but you are not infertile.

Let go of the belief that you are infertile. It is not easy, I understand, but you are in charge of the way you process information that comes to you. So when someone says you are infertile or dealing with infertility, correct them or at least change it in your mind: "No, I may be fertility challenged, but I am preparing my system to become more fertile each day." Ok, this may sound corny but use whatever words make sense to you. I can't say this will reverse menopause and jump start your ovaries if you are over 47 and haven't ovulated in years, but how you respond to people telling you that you are infertile is of the variables you can control to decrease stress on your system to move toward optimizing your fertility.

Certainly, there are those women who aren't producing any eggs and men who aren't producing any sperm, but these situations are the exception, rather than the rule. Remember, even among all the information and statistics, you are an individual, and for the majority of those trying to conceive, it is possible to enhance your fertility by focusing on the steps presented in this book. Feel empowered in the knowledge that this is your body, and you have the power to enhance your overall health and fertility while playing an active role in enhancing your chance to conceive.

3) IVF didn't work for me, so I can't get pregnant.

I can't tell you how many patients have come to me after years of IVF with no results and then become pregnant naturally, or after helping their body recover for at least six months, go on to create pregnancies with procedures that didn't work for them before.

IVF or your response to IVF has very little to do with whether you can become pregnant or not. It has more to do with how you react to the medications and whether the protocol your physician is using is effective for you.

Julie came to me after a tragic accident five years ago. She had lost her husband and three children in a car accident. She woke up one morning and was in a normal marriage with three beautiful children, and a few days later, she was alone.

Thankfully, after a few years of processing intense grief, Julie met someone, and after two years, they married. Though the grief of the tragic episode years earlier will never completely leave her, she was lucky to find love again.

Julie and her new partner wanted to try for children, but with Julie approaching forty-one, the doctor said don't wait, go straight to IVF. So without much preparation, Julie and her new husband embarked on the IVF journey. She thought, well, I never had trouble getting pregnant before, why would I now? She thought IVF was a sure thing.

After taking the medications she did not produce any eggs. Her first attempt was cancelled. She and her husband were devastated.

Doctors told her she was running out of time and she should try again as soon as possible or there wouldn't be much time left.

Julie came to me wanting to start IVF in a couple weeks. Not much I said made her see that it was important to wait and get her body in balance. She went back to IVF after starting a few of the steps from the Five-Step Fertility Solution and she created three eggs and one embryo that was able to be transferred. Unfortunately, it didn't work.

After that, Julie decided to give it six months off and try again. When she came back to see me only a few months later, she was pregnant naturally—now halfway to forty-two—and her pregnancy showed low risk of chromosomal abnormalities. She and her partner were very happy and surprised as well that it could happen naturally. I was surprised that it happened so fast. She went on to have a baby girl.

4) My eggs are too old.

If you read the beginning of this book, you understand that new research has shown that there are stems cells on the outer wall of the ovaries that create oocytes (eggs) each month and there aren't hundreds or thousands of eggs hanging around, getting older by the minute. There is a maturation process of the eggs, just like what happens in every other cell of our body, including the sperm, not to mention, and literally every cell in the body.

As we age and our hormone levels decline, the production of the eggs slow and quality can decrease if health is not a big focus. But thankfully quality can be enhanced as demonstrated by the thousands who have become pregnant following this program.

5) My AMH is too low. I have a low egg count. I have low egg reserve. I am going into menopause and have no or few eggs left.

Also discussed in the beginning of *The Baby Maker's Guide to Becoming Pregnant* is the inaccuracy associated with saying low AMH (Anti-Mullerian Hormone) means you are running out of eggs or that you are knocking on menopause's door.

AMH has doubled and even tripled in patients who have followed the Five-Step Fertility Solution (and normalized in those who started with excessive AMH) but even those who have had low AMH and no change in its level have still gone on to a pregnancy in many cases.

AMH does give you an indication of when you may go into menopause, so if you are forty-four or above, this may be relevant info, but if you are between twenty and forty, it may be years before you run any risk of going into menopause.

6) I am experiencing peri-menopause, so I have to go to IVF right away or I will be in menopause soon and not be able to become pregnant.

Most women can experience perimenopause for up to ten years before they stop ovulating and move into menopause. Peri-menopause is not a fertility death sentence. Women with high FSH on the program have gone on to normalize their FSH levels to be able to conceive naturally or with assistance when other variables were improved.

7) I can't get my wife pregnant.

When the diagnosis of male infertility is given some guys do think that the problem is with them and it's their fault that their wife is not conceiving. Some still tend to not believe it especially if the sperm fertilized the egg with a procedure or if they had children previously.

Having a low sperm count or quality issues can certainly hinder a couple's chance to conceive, but much can be done to improve that scenario.

Much like the man who thinks he doesn't have to do anything to improve the couple's chances of conceiving because his results were normal, a woman whose husband has issues with his sperm shouldn't think there is nothing she can do to improve their situation just because the doctor said her hormones are normal. Both partners working on improving their situation as a couple will significantly improve the relationship and health and wellbeing of each of them, which many times equal improved fertility.

The free fertility tips at naturalfertility.com focus in part on helping you recognize the beliefs and thoughts that you may be experiencing and how to let this "fake news" in your mind go. Remember though, just like the monks who have been meditating for years, if an unwanted thought does come in, that is normal. You won't get rid of these thoughts completely, however you can choose how you respond to them. Do you give power to them by having these thoughts and beliefs as your focus or do you let them go.?

SPECIFIC STEPS TO REDUCE STRESS

Dr. Robert Sapolsky, Princeton professor and author of *Why Zebras Don't Get Ulcers,* suggests three ways to reduce the impact of stress on the body.

They are as follows:

- Eliminate it
- Change your response to it
- Prepare for it

Why Zebras Don't Get Ulcers also discusses how stress hormones can impact the reproductive system. In the short term, Sapolsky explained, stress hormones are "brilliantly adapted" to help you survive an unexpected threat. "You mobilize energy in your thigh muscles, you increase your blood pressure, and you turn off everything that is not essential to surviving, such as digestion, growth, and reproduction," he said. "You think more clearly, and certain aspects of learning and memory are enhanced. All of that is spectacularly adapted if you're dealing with an acute physical stressor."

Non-life-threatening stressors, such as constant worry about relationship issues, fertility issues, deadlines, and so on, can create anxiety and fear. These emotions and the thoughts attached to these emotions trigger the release of cortisol and other stress hormones, which, when consistent, over time, can have devastating consequences to your health. Sapolsky states, "If you turn on the stress response chronically for purely psychological reasons, you increase your risk of adult-onset diabetes and high blood pressure. If you're chronically shutting down the digestive system, there are a bunch of gastrointestinal disorders you're more at risk for, as well."

In children, the continual release of glucocorticoids can suppress the secretion of normal growth hormones. "There's actually a syndrome called stress dwarfism in kids who are so psychologically stressed that growth is markedly impaired," Sapolsky said.

Studies have shown that long-term stress also suppresses the immune system, making you more susceptible to infectious diseases, and can even shut down reproduction by causing erectile dysfunction and disrupting menstrual cycles which can impact fertility.

ELIMINATE THE STRESS

"If something is causing you stress," Dr. Sapolsky says, "eliminate it from your life." Does that mean give up on trying for a baby? Not possible, I hear you say. Thoughts of conceiving permeate every facet of your life.

Think about this step as eliminating the beliefs that are likely false and causing stress (i.e., running out of eggs after thirty-five years old, etc.) and focus on what is possible in the situation.

If you are able, eliminate situations (or people) from your life that cause you stress. If there are people who are causing you unnecessary stress, attempt to decrease or eliminate the stress by communicating with them and coming up with a solution. In some cases such as with family, especially if you have let them know how you feel and their behavior continues, the only solution is avoiding them for a little while or forever.

If one of these people is your spouse then you have a bigger problem on your hands. Seeing a counselor or psychologist to help you work through your issues as a couple can be beneficial. But if your partner won't see a counselor with you, go yourself to get guidance about how you can manage the stress you are experiencing in your relationship.

CHANGE YOUR RESPONSE TO IT

Another way of looking at this step is to shift your focus. Part of this is letting go of the negative emotions attached to fertility issues (or other causes of stress). You may be carrying anger, sadness, fear, and guilt when dealing with fertility issues, all of which in the long term, as Dr. Sapolsky states, can impact your reproductive system if they are your main focus.

It is common to hear about couples giving up or shifting their focus to adopting, and all of a sudden, voila! They are pregnant. Why does that happen? Is it because they stopped thinking about it? Actually, when you speak to these couples, they never completely stopped thinking about it. But they did start shifting their focus to living life, doing a procedure, beginning the adoption process or moving on. Therefore they spend less time focusing on what they lacked and more time focusing on what they could do.

This phenomenon is more common than you think. With the advent of social media, news is more readily available and stories about couples adopting, then learning they were pregnant a short time later, have gone viral. Many of these couples had tried for years to become pregnant, but couldn't. Yet, as soon as they adopted a child, without doing anything different, they were able to conceive naturally without giving it much thought. Coincidence, or rather another example of how shifting your focus can decrease stress on the system and result in a viable pregnancy?

Focus on health

For couples who are trying naturally or with IVF, I suggest you shift your focus to becoming as healthy as possible. Make lifestyle and eating plan changes that can be lifelong and not solely followed only to create a pregnancy.

Live your life.

So many couples put their life on hold when trying to conceive. They might stay in a job they hate and tell themselves, "When I become pregnant, I can quit," or "I can use all my sick leave and holiday pay, so I have to stay until I am pregnant."

If a pregnancy doesn't occur for a few years, going to a job every day that you hate just adds more stress to your system and can make it more difficult to conceive.

Samantha was working in a job that she despised. When I asked her why, she said she was saving up her vacation days for maternity leave. I asked her if she knew for sure that her long hours and stress from work were contributing to her not conceiving, would she consider looking for other employment? She looked at me as if a lightbulb went on and said, "Of course I would, if that were the reason I wasn't conceiving." I didn't need to say any more. At an office visit a short time later, Samantha told me she was pregnant with her first child. I was surprised it happened so quickly and asked if she changed jobs.

"No, not yet," she responded. "It seemed like just knowing that I could change and then starting the process of looking helped me reduce my stress. I wasn't as depressed or anxious going to work anymore because I knew I was eventually not going to be there much longer. I stopped letting all the stuff get to me."

Are you avoiding going on a holiday or doing something you would enjoy because you are afraid you may be pregnant?

Marie had two teenage children from a previous marriage when she came to us. She had been trying to conceive with her new partner, but it just was not happening. After she and her partner were on the program for six months and nothing was happening, though all tests and his semen analysis looked good, I asked if she had room in her life for another child. It seemed that she was always busy running around, complaining how little time she had to do temperatures and see the doctor. She was stressed out and felt she had no time left. Together, we looked at her life and what she could do differently. What stress relieving activities could she do? Marie told me she used to love spending time with her teenagers, going on hikes, and playing polo at the club.

When I asked why she hadn't done those activities recently, her answer was, "I don't have time, and I wouldn't want to ride a horse in case I fell off and I was pregnant." It turned out she had forgotten how much she really loved the time spent playing polo with her teens.

The next time we talked, Marie seemed like a different person. She was back to hiking on the weekends instead of bringing work home, and once a week she was playing polo again. They had also planned a family ski trip, as well. After that visit, I hadn't heard from Marie for more than a year, but I received a card in the mail that was a baby announcement. She had become pregnant on their family ski trip and couldn't have been happier, but she had been so busy she forgot to tell me.

Do you have to quit your job, go skiing, and start playing polo to get pregnant? No, not exactly.

What you can do is stop putting your life on hold. Find a good balance.

Work-life balance is a bit of a misnomer though. Work is a part of our life so do we really want to consider work outside of our life. That certainly won't make Monday mornings any easier.

Instead just consider 'life balance." Create a plan about what you can do to balance your health and wellbeing at work and outside of work. Whatever you do, get out of a job that you hate or have a plan to do so to open up possibilities for yourself. Find a balance that you can healthily maintain without thinking "But what if I get pregnant?" Remember, you have to live life in order to receive it.

Prepare Yourself for It

It is interesting that most people spend so much time and energy trying *not* to get pregnant for so many years and really do not do much usually to prepare themselves to become pregnant.

Based on what we know about follicular development (Stanford University has shown that the human follicle can take up to eight menstrual cycles to develop before it ever comes up on the ovary, 2000), the egg is developing at least from day one of the cycle to ovulation, and the sperm can take up to three months to regenerate.

Preparation is key to creating a healthy, viable embryo.

Preparation, however, is what so many couples skip because due to pressure from themselves, family, the media or the medical profession, they feel they need to rush into the procedure because time is running out. For the first year of trying, many people go to their doctors and hear, "Don't worry, it hasn't been twelve months yet. Most couples conceive within twelve months, so if it hasn't happened by then, come back, and we will look into it."

This is a frustrating response for most because they often want to be able to do something to help improve their chances. Because of that drive the next step is scour the internet for information to help them while pretending not to worry about it.

Then when the couple or the female comes back at twelve months and one day, usually some tests are done, and drugs like Clomiphene are administered without looking at diet or lifestyle, stress levels, and so on. If Clomiphene doesn't work, then they are told to try insemination, and if that doesn't work, then off to IVF. These days if you are over thirty-five they often skip clomid and insemination and recommend IVF right away without any preparation at all.

So empowering yourself and preparing your body are often skipped until none of the medical intervention works. That often results in a lot of anguish from the emotional and financial toll that procedures can have on the system and the pocketbook. Then as you try to improve your health, you feel you are constantly working against time and don't have enough time to prepare. It is a vicious cycle that just promotes more stress *unless* you follow the steps in this book and focus on what is possible.

Healthcare professionals miss an important opportunity during that first twelve months of trying to help their patients become educated in some of the most basic steps to optimizing their chance to conceive, and by the time they go into IVF, most do not understand what the drugs are doing and do not get themselves emotionally or physically prepared for the procedure and pregnancy.

Jackie's story is very typical of most. "It felt like a whirlwind," she says. "We were convinced that after a year of trying and then using Clomid that IVF was finally the answer. We were going to be pregnant. Then after time went on and we had five fresh attempts with no explanation of why it didn't work, I came up for air."

"Hormones were in overdrive from the medications and just took over. I never considered taking time to step back and prepare my body for this procedure. The emphasis was on urgency. I was thirty-seven when we started, and according to the doctors, this was over the hill as far as fertility was concerned. I couldn't believe how much time had passed with me doing the same thing over and over again and foolishly expecting a different result."

This is very common among people who visit an IVF clinic without focusing on the many areas they can address before moving to an assisted procedure. After visiting an IVF clinic and being told the clock is ticking, you are running out of time, it's easy to focus on the fear related to the perception of "running out of eggs" or the "biological clock is ticking." It is easy to fall into this trap, but preparation in many cases is the key to creating a viable pregnancy naturally or with a procedure.

You can prepare yourselves physically by following the Five-Step Fertility Solution™. You can prepare yourselves physiologically by taking time to understand the process, understanding that your body takes time to improve and balance itself, and addressing stress through counseling, reading the fertility tips on our website, and from meditation, workshops, and asking for support from those you love.

Realize that your fertility won't go away in a few months' time. There is not some cliff that one day your body falls off into the oblivion of menopause. The exception to this rule is if your body experience extreme stress in a short period of time, i.e. chemotherapy, radiation, a sudden and impactful loss, etc. The majority of the time your body just simply does not work that way. Moving into the next phase of life takes time. Perimenopause, the period of time before menopause when a woman can still become pregnant, can last for ten years or more. The average age of menopause is 50.5, and you can still technically conceive up until then. I have worked with women who were forty-seven and forty-eight conceive with their own eggs naturally and with IVF.

FERTILITY OVER FORTY

Jane was forty-four when she started the program. She had been trying for six years and had several IVF procedures. When she started, she had committed to taking twelve months off treatment, even though her doctors thought she was crazy.

She addressed all the areas that I discuss in this book. She and her husband took the five steps to a new level, and returned to IVF at forty-five. Doctors told her it would never happen and gave her a less than a 1 percent chance.

In her next fresh cycle, she and her partner created the most embryos they ever had, but the fresh cycle didn't work. She did, however, have frozen embryos from this fresh cycle that she could use later. Jane took a further three months to prepare for the frozen cycle. Her doctors now told her the chance was even less and that no one her age had ever conceived from a frozen embryo in their country. Well, Jane beat the odds and had a baby girl from the frozen embryo transfer at forty-five years of age after taking one year off to prepare.

Jane's story illustrates how important it is to prepare yourself physiologically and emotionally for your procedures. Jane said she never had felt as balanced as she did going through the fresh cycle, and she wasn't deflated when the fresh cycle did not work. She had a sense that she was going to be okay, no matter what happened.

COMMUNICATION

One major source of stress with couples as they are continuing along their fertility journey is relationship stress. Fertility issues tend to either bring a couple much closer together, or if you aren't proactive by practicing upfront healthy communication, the stress of the fertility journey can drive some couples apart. It will also exacerbate the issues in a relationship that was already rocky.

At times, one spouse can be very adamant about doing everything possible to conceive, while the other says, "If it is meant to be, it will just happen."

These two opposite attitudes, when dealing with fertility issues, can be a source of great stress and leaves both people feeling separate, disconnected, and many times angry, fearful, and depressed.

Consistent communication is the key. Remember these points when tension gets high and uncomfortable:

1. Don't expect your spouse to react the same way as you do.

   As humans, we react differently to stress. Just because he isn't crying like you are, it doesn't mean he doesn't care. Just because she is crying more than usual, doesn't mean she is being too emotional. Understand that you will both deal with this crisis in your own unique way.

2. Keep the channels of communication open.

   Let your partner know how you feel, and ask them to respect those feelings even if that is not the way he/she is seeing the situation. Ask for their help, support, and understanding.

3. Tell them what you want them to do.

   When you are crying, do you just want them to hold you tight? When you are angry, do you just want to be left alone? Remember the one line I like from Dr. Phil, "Teach people how to treat you." If they don't respond or listen, get outside help and support from a counselor or therapist.

4. When the feelings are less intense or not at their extreme, talk to each other. Avoid bringing the sensitive topics up right before a period, or when you are supposed to time intercourse. Find time away from those heightened times of stress to talk about what is going on.

   For her: Don't expect him to go deeply into his feelings about the situation. Think about what he could do to help you and communicate this to him so if you fall in a heap or have a bad day, he knows what to do.

   For him: Expect her to feel this deeply and be afraid. She needs your support, but she knows you can't fix it for her. Tell her if you are feeling pressure to perform, and let her know if you feel as though she doesn't respond to you intimately, unless it's baby-making time.

5. Make time to connect to each other outside of the baby-making window.

   Have a few date nights a month, and make an effort to have a few romantic evenings. Spend that time talking about how you are feeling about your fertility issues, but give that a time limit, and make sure you talk about how you can start to live life again.

6. Show your partner you appreciate him/her.

   Make a list each day of three things you appreciate about your spouse, and show him or her one night or surprise him or her with it on a sticky note in the car, on the bathroom mirror, or on their pillow before he or she go to bed.

7. Seek out a relationship counselor who can help you communicate better by showing you how to understand your partner's way of communicating.

   Sometimes when a person is more visual, he or she communicate better when you show them what you need. If a visual person can <u>see</u> why it is important to you, it may help him or her understand your needs better. Others are more kinesthetic and may need to get <u>a feel</u> for it or understand more through doing, role playing, or through a physical connection such as a hand on their arm when you are talking or holding hands to make a physical kinesthetic connection. Some people understand better just by being spoken to. They tend to learn more easily through sound or voice. The auditory person will relate to what it <u>sounds</u> like more than seeing or feeling why something is important.

8. Communicate to your spouse using his or her communication style, not yours.

   If you use your communication style, your spouse will be less likely to understand what you mean and how you are feeling. Are they visual, kinesthetic, or auditory? Do they make comments such as "I <u>see</u> what you mean." "I <u>hear</u> what you are saying." "I have <u>this feeling</u> you don't understand me." Speak to them with their communication style. It will feel odd and even contrived at first, but you will have a much better chance of getting their attention.

   Turn to the free fertility tips on our website to understand how to identify your communication style and your partner's and tips on how you can communicate more effectively.

Find out what works for you as a couple. Relationships are not easy to maintain and require constant attention. Despite the pain you are experiencing regarding fertility issues, remind yourself why you married this person. Use that as your motivation to reconnect and communicate effectively.

If you try to find support in your spouse but that person for whatever reason does not give you the support that you feel you need, then reach out and create a support system of friends and family or a professional support system that you can go to when you need someone to be there through the tough times. Confide in someone close that you trust so you do not feel alone. It is your responsibility to reach out for help when you need it. People are so busy with their own stuff these days and couples tend to keep fertility issues to themselves. Your friends and family may not know you need help. Reach out and let them know how they can help you.

HELP IS OUT THERE

If you are looking for help, you need to find the program that fits you. Letting go of any fear, anger, or guilt that may surround fertility issues can create amazing results.

When looking for a program whether it is a counselor, physician or holistic health professional, I would suggest the following:

- Make sure the person you want to work with has experience working with couples dealing with fertility issues.
- Make sure you feel comfortable and congruent with the people you are working with. Ask them questions about their experience with other couples. Ask them what the three most important things you can do to improve your situation. If these things ring true or if they help you come up with your own answer, then you have probably found someone you will feel empowered to work with.

- Understand that no one is going to fix you and that it is important to take responsibility and become an active participant in improving your emotional wellbeing.
- Be kind to yourself in the process.

I know reaching out for help is easier said than done when dealing with fertility issues, but utilizing counseling, workshops, or techniques such as timeline therapy technique, hypnotherapy, emotional freedom technique, or more traditional cognitive behavioral therapy with a psychologist who specializes in this area, you can work on eliminating the beliefs that are causing daily stressors on your system.

I sincerely believe mind-body connection is one of the most important areas and is key to improving a couple's situation.

My *Get Off the Emotional Rollercoaster* recording is available at the membership site for patients at www.tipstogetpregnant.com. This has helped many couples remind themselves of what is possible in a society focused on limitations. E-mail info@naturalfertility.com if you want more information on how to become a member of this site. Ask for the special *Baby Maker's Guide* discount an and a free copy of How to Get Off the Emotional Rollercoaster recording will be sent to you.

GRIEVING YOUR PERCEIVED LOSS EACH MONTH

The following is a fertility tip I sent out a few years ago and still send out once a year because it seems to strike a chord with many who are dealing with fertility issues.

A few years ago, a dear friend of mine lost her child in a car accident to a drunken driver. Her son was only six years old. It was an extremely sad story. I watched my friend go through all the stages of grieving, and she certainly had her good days, along with the bad days. During this time, as I observed all the stages of grieving with my friend, it dawned on me, "This is what many of my patients go through every month."

Not sure what I mean? Let's discuss the stages of grieving. There are five stages in the grieving process. According to Dr. Elizabeth

Kubler Ross, who was a guru on the topic of grieving, the five stages are as follows:

1. Denial
2. Depression
3. Anger
4. Bargaining
5. Acceptance

How do these stages apply to you?

Denial

Do you ever get a few cramps or heaviness in your lower abdomen right before your period starts? Maybe when that headache occurs or the breast soreness starts, the little voice in the back of your mind may be saying, "Well, maybe that's not my period; maybe I could be pregnant." After all, you timed intercourse correctly, everyone is telling you to stop worrying about it, it will just happen, and yep, this could be the month.

Depression

Or when those symptoms begin, you begin to slide into sadness or depression but grip onto the one glimmer of hope that the period hasn't started quite yet, so maybe this time you are pregnant (denial again). Then a few days later, the period starts, and you feel deflated and depressed as if someone has pulled the carpet out from under you both, punched you in the stomach, or somehow defeated you again.

Everything seemed right that month. What am I or what are we doing wrong? What is wrong with me/us? Sadness and depression, even *anger*, set in.

Next thing you know, the period is in full swing. The temperatures have dropped, and you come to *accept* that you aren't pregnant. Once again, it's time to start all over.

This time you think, "I will eat better, exercise more, and stay on track this cycle. I know if I do this, then maybe it will happen this month, right? If only it could happen this month. I will go to church every Sunday and be the best person I can be, if only it could happen this month." (*Bargaining*).

Or you may think, "What's the use? One more beer, one more wine won't hurt. See, I told you giving up the cigarettes last month, the coffee, the wine, and the chocolate wouldn't make a difference. What's the use?" (*Anger* or *apathy*).

Ovulation approaches, and you know it's time for baby-making again. You have reluctantly been charting your temperatures now, and you can tell ovulation is nearly here.

At times, you both look at each other thinking "Not again." You almost begin to dread what should be intimate loving (or at least fun) moments, but you know if you want a child, it has to be done. Your attitude toward sex is significantly different than before you started baby-making, that's for sure!

You might think, "If we only knew it was going to be this hard back then, we wouldn't have tried so hard *not* to get pregnant."

A fight may break out right around ovulation, or you might have no sex drive whatsoever. After intercourse, if you had it, the glimmer of hope returns; and though you try to push it away, you try to hide it, that little voice in the back of your mind keeps whispering "Maybe this month."

The two weeks pass while you try your best not to pay attention to every twinge and every sensation that you feel in your body (which is now magnified by about two thousand times). Could I/she be pregnant?

Bargaining can come into play here again. You may even make a promise to God or the universe that if it happens this month, you will pray more, spend more time with the disadvantaged, strive to be the best parent you can be, stop being so crabby, have a normal happy life. You promise to be a better person. If only you could be pregnant, everything else would be okay.

Have you felt this way ever? Had any of these thoughts or feelings? Gone through any of these stages?

If you have, you are certainly not alone. It's very common. Whether you or your spouse experience just one of these thoughts or many remember you are not alone.

This grieving process that you may go through each month may take its toll, but at some point, just like when you have lost a person you love, there comes a time when focusing on the loss makes you stop living, and it becomes time once again for the loss to change to appreciation of life. First start with your own. Appreciate the life you have, instead of focusing on what you lack.

The process of grieving the loss of a loved one can be complete at some point because you have (hopefully) the good memories to focus on. But grieving the loss of something you haven't had is a grueling process because there doesn't seem to be a beginning, middle, or end. There are no memories to cherish, only pain to experience each month. This is not a healthy or happy existence. However, you have the ability to stop this cycle and live life to receive it.

Shifting the focus to what you have is the key. This doesn't take the desire to have a baby away, and it certainly doesn't mean that you won't at any moment welcome a baby into your life. It only makes the waiting and preparing more bearable, more productive, and more purposeful until it happens for you.

Is It Time to Draw the Line?

There may be a time, if it doesn't happen for you, that you decide to draw the line because you know you have done everything in your power and that you have left no stone unturned to help make it happen.

At that time, hopefully, you have done the one thing that you may have forgotten about until right now, and that is no matter what happens, you have accepted yourself as the worthwhile and beautiful person that you are right this minute, with a child or without one. At the end of the day, that is true acceptance.

Toni understands what true acceptance really means. She came to the clinic for eight months, trying to become pregnant after nine years of trying. She had set a deadline of six months to conceive but extended that to a year after the six month mark came and went.

However, at eight months, she came into my office with a smile on her face, and I was ready to hear that she was pregnant, but that is not what she told me. She said that even though she was feeling good on the program and her health had never been better, she and her partner, Jarrod, decided it was time to draw the line. She wanted to continue eating healthy and stay on herbs and supplements for her general well being because her energy with her period had improved. She wasn't feeling any PMS. And the cramping had also disappeared, but she was ready to stop trying and just live her life to the fullest.

Toni continued on the program to keep her healthy, and we decided I would see her in six months' time to see how she was doing. The first visit after that appointment, I asked her how she was coping, and she replied, "Great. Your fertility tips helped me a great deal. I realized that I needed to live my life and let go of all the guilt and shame along with the expectations of having my own child. I am blessed that with my job, I get to see children every day and try to positively influence their lives. I realized that was enough for me and that I married my partner for him, not just so we could have kids. I know in my heart this is the right path for us." She went on to say, "I absolutely adore my nieces and really enjoy the time I spend with them, when before while I was trying, I realized I was actually avoiding them."

"Our lives are full now, and though we have our challenges, we are not looking back with regret."

I continue to see Toni in consultations six months to twelve months to check in on how she is doing with her overall health and wellbeing. She never got pregnant but found other ways to appreciate what she was truly accomplishing by contributing to children's lives every day. She felt good moving forward with her life.

BE AT PEACE

Whether you are deciding to draw the line or you are continuing to do everything you can possibly do to create the life that you long for, accepting you and your partner for who you are, not defining yourself by what you don't have, is the path that will bring life to you in the most amazing, unexpected, and fulfilling ways. For some, it brings children and all the wonderful and challenging times they bring. For others, like Toni, she realized what her path was meant to be and pursued happiness and joy in her life. Most of all, whether you continue to do everything you possibly can to have a child or you decide to draw the line, knowing that you will be okay no matter what will bring you true peace and acceptance. Whatever path you take, this is truly what I hope for you.

WHAT YOUR DOCTOR MAY NOT HAVE TOLD YOU ABOUT YOUR FERTILITY

WHEN I GIVE talks online or in person some people say, I fixed my diet. I take a prenatal vitamin, I am not really that stressed. So I am doing all the things you are talking about and I am still not pregnant. Why?

Well, when I sit down with these individuals or couples it becomes apparent that they aren't doing all of the five steps together at the same time. Fixing the diet is more than simply cutting out carbs. As discussed in the Baby Maker's Guide to Getting Pregnant, often-times you need more than a prenatal. And what about exercise and minimizing toxins? Addressing these steps and managing stress is imperative to increasing your chances.

Make sure you are applying the steps in detail (not just one step for x amount of time and another step for x amount of time) together to get the best results.

But I am going to give you the benefit of the doubt. Let's say you are truly applying all five steps all the time. What do you do if it is still not happening?

This chapter, "What Your Doctor May Not Have Told You about Your Fertility," may help you find the answers that you are looking for.

FEELING HELPLESS?

When couples are told that everything is fine and there is no appar-ent reason why they cannot conceive, why they keep miscarrying, or why even though they have a diagnosis, all the medications and procedures didn't work… it is beyond frustrating.

Their doctors perform tests and determine that everything looks okay—there simply aren't any additional identifiable medical issues to explain why they cannot create a viable pregnancy. They are left feeling helpless. They are told it must be their age, or just to keep trying whether it be another procedure, another month on Clomid or to take a vacation and stop thinking about it.

With no answers from their general practitioners or family medicine doctors, they turn to fertility specialists for procedures in the hopes of improving their chances and or complementary medicine clinics for insight if the medical system doesn't work for them.

Kay is a great example. She and her partner came in to see me after being told there was no apparent reason for their fertility issues. They were told the next step was IVF. Kay was twenty-eight at the time, and her partner was in his early thirties. They didn't want to do IVF right away due to the expense, and to them, it seemed strange to spend money on a procedure when no one was able to tell them why they weren't becoming pregnant.

After reading through their information and test results, nothing jumped out as a big issue. There was, however, mention of some irritable bowel symptoms occasionally and regular bloating following meals. With this information, I generally ask for more specific blood tests that haven't been done yet and begin addressing the digestive symptoms. After all, as you now know, if the gut isn't working, then nutrients may not be getting absorbed optimally. Therefore, the health of the cells, including the eggs and sperm, may suffer.

Kay returned to her next appointment after consistently using the herbs and supplements. Her new blood tests didn't reveal much more than her first set, but one thing did jump out at me. Her digestive symptoms did not improve at all. The bloating continued, and the symptoms that had been diagnosed as irritable bowel syndrome in the past were back.

This made me wonder a bit more about her gut health, and I asked her to discuss this with her doctor having one more test done to assess whether she there was indication of an intolerance to gluten or what is commonly known as celiac disease.

When Kay returned for her next visit, she had the biggest smile on her face. I thought for sure she was pregnant, but she wasn't. When she sat down, she threw her arms in the air and said, "I have celiac disease!" I have never seen someone so happy to be diagnosed with gluten intolerance. She felt so much relief that they finally found a possible cause for why they hadn't been becoming pregnant.

Kay told me about her conversation with her doctor before she had the test done. The doctor told Kay there was no way that she had celiac disease, but they would order the test anyway to put her mind at ease. Well, the test came back positive, showing elevated antibodies and confirming her probable intolerance to gluten. The only way they could say without a doubt that she had celiac disease was with a gastroscopy or endoscopy. This is where a camera is put down your throat and goes through your stomach to your small intestine to see if there is evidence of damage to structures called villi. This is a tell-tale sign of gluten intolerance. Kay decided to forgo the test and just avoid gluten. Seven weeks after going gluten free, Kay rang in to say that she was pregnant. This story has repeated itself over and over through the years with different couples.

Celiac disease is not the answer for everyone dealing with fertility issues, but Kay's story illustrates that when the doctor says all tests have been done that could possibly be done, this doesn't mean there are not tests left to do. Instead, it means the cause hasn't been found...yet based on the testing they have done. This chapter will address the most commonly overlooked issues for couples dealing with fertility issues who despite having all tests come up normal are still not pregnant or who have had confirmed diagnosis such as polycystic ovaries (PCOS), endometriosis, fibroids, or recurrent miscarriage and a viable pregnancy still eludes them.

One of our goals is to identify factors that may contribute to difficulty conceiving.

Let me say at the outset that I am not against medical doctors, and I always strive to create a team approach when assisting any couple. Whenever a doctor is willing, we work with them. It is our belief that fostering this relationship can only be beneficial for the couple and the focus should always be on supporting the couple as best as possible.

Our approach looks at some of the factors involved with fertility issues that are sometimes ignored or not considered important or credible by mainstream medicine.

In diagnosing a fertility issue, physicians typically will evaluate the woman extensively and order lab tests that typically rule out sexual transmitted diseases, make sure their immunity in some areas is intact, and attempt to make sure she is ovulating. If the woman is over thirty-five, they do one or two tests to check if she is in menopause. For the man, the tests are much less involved and usually only a semen analysis is performed, despite the fact that best medical practices say the male should have two or three semen analysis to assess his situation. The results of the evaluation and tests can lead them to a diagnosis. However, there are times when routine tests come back within normal range. If everything else looks fine, there is nothing to base the cause of their fertility on, therefore resulting in the diagnosis of unexplained fertility—or if there is a diagnosis, then "we really don't know why you aren't getting pregnant," followed by "your eggs may be too old." Unfortunately, too many people accept this diagnosis and think there is nothing they can do. Worse still, the woman often bears the brunt of the guilt for waiting too long to have a baby. She can be twenty-five or forty-five and hear the news that her eggs aren't healthy or are too old. Yet there is no test that gives confirmation or credibility to these statements. That is truly a guess, because there is no perfectly reliable diagnostic test to say this in fact is true

NORMAL RANGE IS *NOT* ENOUGH

"But my doctor says everything is normal", is a statement I hear from almost every new patient that I see. When lab results are within normal range, it means they are within the average range often for the population being tested. Normal ranges are not "healthy" ranges. But when everything is normal or a person is on medication to make everything look normal, and a viable pregnancy isn't happening the next step is medication, insemination or IVF. However, in my experience, it has become apparent that normal test results are not always optimal for pregnancy.

First, most lab results are read and interpreted according to preset ranges, with a low and a high number indicating the limits based on a certain population. Therefore normal is often based on population normal and anything that falls within that range.

If you ask your local pathology scientists if the normal ranges on the medical test results represent healthy ranges, they will tell you "no." Most of these ranges represent the average in a population.

Is it simply okay to be within the range, or is it preferable or a problem to be at the upper or lower end? These are questions that must be explored when addressing fertility issues because if everything was truly normal or optimal for pregnancy, you probably wouldn't need to read this book. More times than not, there are variables that aren't being addressed or assessed when everything appears normal.

It's also true that what is considered <u>abnormal</u> for one laboratory testing facility may actually be <u>normal</u> in another. The standard ranges vary from one facility to another. In fact, I've seen lab results for couples that fall within the normal range on per one lab, but the results would be considered abnormal at another lab. This raises additional questions and warrants further investigation when supporting a couple trying to conceive.

If what is considered normal ranges from a low to a high, and if there are different medical opinions on what is normal versus what is abnormal, it becomes obvious that normal has too many variables. The truth is what is considered to be normal in the medical industry might not be optimal for conception for everyone. For that reason, my clinic has been assessing blood results for hundred women and men every year who were able to create a live birth from 2005 to 2014. I received copies of lab results from the first time they saw me, and approximately every three months after that until the time they conceived. I took the levels closest to pregnancy and averaged them to find out our "optimal levels". Therefore we went from looking at several different populations to what the levels on average were for women who were becoming pregnant with viable pregnancies while on our program.

Important information is often missed when relying solely on the normal ranges. When addressing fertility issues, better results are consistently created when results are in the optimal range.

For these reasons, it becomes apparent simply relying on "everything looks normal" will end up contributing to them falling short of creating a viable pregnancy. The less than optimal levels may give clues the other factors that aren't being addressed. The good news is that many of these contributing factors to fertility issues can be identified and addressed.

More good news is that the medical community is beginning to recognize this at least for some test results and fertility. For example, thyroid function, which we will talk about later, may be normal by medical standards but currently there is evidence that if one of the test results for thyroid function is within an optimal range, the person has a better chance of a procedure creating a viable pregnancy. More on this later in this chapter.

Let's start with what we see to be a subtle, yet significant, part of dealing with fertility issues—the delicate balance of hormones in the body.

HORMONAL BALANCE IS KEY

The balance of estrogen and progesterone is a good example of an often overlooked and completely ignored facet of women's fertility. Medical professionals do not usually recognize the significance of the balance between estrogen and progesterone largely because there is not much consensus in mainstream medicine on what constitutes the optimal balance between these two hormones.

Based on thousands of couples I have seen over the years, we have identified a range of what we consider the optimal hormone balance between these hormones at certain stages in the female reproductive cycle. However, this range is not set in stone. Each person is an individual. Therefore, their individual situation should be considered along with tests, reports, and symptoms.

At my clinic, I used our optimal range as a guideline or an indication of where to go from there. Practitioners that are a part of my Baby Maker Network, a certification program that focuses on training practitioners how to effectively apply the Five-Step Fertility Solution and dive deeply into the assessment of couples fertility issues, are very familiar with these ranges and how to apply them.

Certain diagnoses can give the practitioner clues as to whether a person may be suffering from less than optimal hormone balance. This less than optimal balance is often represented as estrogen dominance, where the balance between estrogen and progesterone is not optimal.

ESTROGEN DOMINANCE

Estrogen dominance occurs when estrogen (usually estradiol when dealing with fertility issues) is out of balance with the hormone progesterone. Estrogen may be too high compared to normal or low progesterone or progesterone may be low in comparison to normal or high estrogen. Another hormone estrone can also contribute to estrogen dominance so this should be investigated if estradiol seems low but symptoms of estrogen dominance still exist.

The following list represents some common symptoms of estrogen dominance:

Women

- Weight gain with your period or around ovulation due to fluid retention or bloating/swelling of the abdomen.
- Premenstrual tension including irritability, sugar cravings
- Migraines or headaches around ovulation, before or during menses
- Cramping, pain, or bloating around ovulation
- Endometriosis
- Ovarian cysts
- Fibroids
- Sore, swollen breasts leading up to the period, with period, or at ovulation
- Tender or swollen nipples leading up to period, with period or at ovulation
- Cervical dysplasia (CIN)
- Breast, cervical, or uterine cancer
- Acne at ovulation, or leading up to or during period
- Spotting leading up to period or after

Men

- Prostate issues
- Low sperm count (not conclusive but noted as a probable factor in overweight men who have low sperm count)
- Breast formation often referred to as "Man Boobs"

Note: These symptoms can be common with other issues as well so investigation by your practitioner is necessary to differentiate the potential cause(s)

CAUSES OF ESTROGEN DOMINANCE
EXCESS ESTROGEN

Estrogen dominance can occur in women and men for various reasons. In some women, estrogen dominance can be due to long-term use of the pill or synthetic estrogen medications.

Depending on the individual, why they went on the pill in the first place, and whether they were experiencing estrogen dominance before starting the pill, long-term use of the pill in some women can also lead to continued imbalance between estrogen and progesterone.

Another less recognized cause of estrogen dominance in both men and women is the exposure to xeno-estrogens, which are environmental chemicals with the ability to mimic estrogen in your body. Unfortunately, there are too many situations when we are unknowingly exposed to these types of endocrine disruptors that impact your fertility.

Exposure to xeno-estrogens can come from cooking in plastic containers in the microwave. Other sources as discussed in The Baby Maker's Guide To Getting Pregnant are paper carryout cups at the café, receipts, plastic water bottles, skin care products, processed foods, and some pesticides, herbicides, dyes, and preservatives.

PROGESTERONE DEFICIENCY

Estrogen is not always the only issue when looking at the optimal balance of progesterone and estrogen. Progesterone deficiency is often the issue and can also be referred to as estrogen dominance even when estrogen is in the optimal range. If progesterone isn't sufficient enough to combat the effects of estrogen even when estrogen is normal then a person is likely to experience the symptoms of estrogen dominance. Estrogen is a proliferative hormone. That means it makes things grow such as the females eggs up to ovulation and breast tissue, especially if not balanced by progesterone in the luteal phase leading up to the period. Cysts can also be an issue with deficient progesterone or excessive estrogen.

Progesterone helps balance the effects of estrogen. For example, estrogen begins the thickening of the uterine lining in the first half of the menstrual cycle and progesterone finishes it off in the luteal phase making the lining more receptive to the implantation of an embryo. Scientists Groothuis and Dassen from the Netherlands state: "Once the functional layer has successfully been rebuilt (by estrogen), the actions of progesterone change the estrogen primed endometrium into a receptive state." (Source: *Human Reproduction*, 2007)

When we refer to progesterone deficiency, we refer to low levels of progesterone that may not be sufficient to create a healthy lining of the uterus necessary for implantation. Because the follicle that carries the egg produces the progesterone after the egg's release (which is then referred to as the corpus luteum), if progesterone is low, we have to question the health of the follicle and potentially the health of the egg it released.

CAUSES OF PROGESTERONE DEFICIENCY

Low progesterone commonly occurs in times of increased stress when the body converts progesterone into cortisol due to prolonged stress.

The stress response otherwise known as fight or flight response of our bodies typically alters reproductive hormonal output. Since the adrenals regulate this response and when under stress are continually stimulated due to physiological or emotional stress, this can decrease the chance for a conception to occur or a pregnancy to be maintained if this stress effects progesterone levels. Progesterone can actually be converted into cortisol during high or prolonged periods of stress, instead of being optimized for fertility purposes. Stress can be emotional or solely physiological such as stress resulting from chemical exposure, food sensitivities, the flu, increased inflammation for a poor diet, etc.

If the corpus luteum (the leftover follicle) is faulty or small and does not produce enough progesterone, the message to and from the pituitary may not occur properly, and progesterone production could be diminished. If the luteal phase, or second half of the cycle, is short (i.e., less than fourteen days), this can be due to low progesterone and is referred to as a luteal phase defect or luteal phase insufficiency. This situation is often related to problems with implantation.

If a person has a fourteen-day or normal-length luteal phase but the progesterone is low, this could be due to stress and the adrenals as mentioned, as well as less than optimal thyroid function. Thyroid hormones help stimulate progesterone production, so if the thyroid hormones are less than optimal, progesterone may be less than optimal as well.

Let's examine some of the common symptoms you may experience with progesterone deficiency.

SYMPTOMS OF PROGESTERONE DEFICIENCY (CAN ALSO BE REFERRED TO AS ESTROGEN DOMINANCE)

- Hormonal acne
- Depression
- Bloating before or during your period
- Breast tenderness
- Premenstrual headaches
- Spotty or scanty periods smoke
- Spotting leading up to period
- Short luteal phase (second half of cycle is shorter than fourteen days)
- Any premenstrual symptoms
- Fibroids

- Endometriosis
- Ovarian Cysts

> Note: Many of the symptoms above are experienced with estrogen dominance because, as discussed, progesterone deficiency can be why estrogen, even at normal levels, is dominant.

If you are wondering whether progesterone deficiency is an issue you can find clues on your temperature charts. If your temperature chart does not show a sustained rise in temperature after ovulation this may indicate progesterone is an issue. You may also notice your temperature (and possibly progesterone) dropping in and out throughout the luteal phase (second half of the cycle after ovulation). This can indicate that your body is trying to secrete progesterone but may not be maintaining the levels necessary for an adequate endometrial lining (lining of the uterus) throughout the luteal phase. Temperature charts cannot tell us the actual level of progesterone however and therefore it is necessary to check progesterone levels in comparison to estrogen with other objective data seven days after ovulation. These tests can be done through saliva or blood testing.

At least 70–80 percent of women who present as patients in my clinic present with progesterone levels lower than the optimal range when I first see them.

As stated above, blood tests seven days after ovulation for estradiol and progesterone can give you an idea if progesterone levels are less than optimal. But unfortunately many doctors will send patients for their progesterone test on day twenty-one of their cycle without ever asking them how long their cycle is. Day twenty-one is perfect if you have a twenty-eight days cycle because day twenty-one is seven days after likely ovulation (day fourteen) of a twenty-eight day cycle. But if your cycle isn't always twenty-eight days, then doing a day twenty-one test can be inaccurate and lead your physician to the wrong conclusion. You could be told you aren't ovulating when you just hadn't ovulated yet. For example if your cycles are thirty-six days, to figure out probable ovulation, you would subtract fourteen from your cycle length because that is the usual length of the luteal phase. Therefore thirty-six minus fourteen is twenty-two. If you test on day twenty-one, you wouldn't have ovulated yet. If your cycle is short, that is twenty-four days, then probable ovulation would be day ten (twenty-four days minus fourteen equals ten). If you test on day twenty-one, that is only a few days before your period is due and progesterone may be lower because your period is coming on. Always test the balance of estrogen and progesterone seven days post ovulation. How to track ovulation is discussed in chapter 3, "Determining Ovulation."

HORMONE CREAMS: TOO MUCH OF A GOOD THING?

If progesterone is too low, it seems the logical next step would be to take progesterone to attempt to increase the hormone in the system. However taking progesterone does not address the reason why progesterone was low. Therefore, adrenal or thyroid issues will continue to impact hormone balance, and though progesterone may be increased in the short term and you may find short term relief of symptoms, adding progesterone over the long term may end up causing an imbalance if not properly monitored. I see this mostly when patients are using progesterone cream long term without the person who prescribed it to them following up with saliva tests. Blood tests are not valid when using progesterone cream due to the progesterone bypassing the stomach and going right into the tissues from the skin. Blood tests only measure what is floating around in the blood, not what is already absorbed and acting on the tissues.

The same tends to be true for progesterone suppositories or pessaries, and progesterone injections. If you are taking progesterone orally blood tests have some value but our ultimate goal is to see if progesterone is getting absorbed into the tissue and blood tests are not a good indicator of how much hormone has gotten into the tissue. For this reason saliva testing is often preferred.

Some women swear by hormone creams, which I completely understand because when they start using them, they often feel much better. Symptoms decrease or disappear and they feel they have found the answer to their problems. Some women actually become pregnant after using progesterone.

However, I would advise exercising caution when using hormone creams because it isn't addressing the cause of the issue and overdosing the tissue with hormones is a common problem. If your body is getting too much of a hormone, then it will slow down its production of that hormone. So long term use of progesterone not properly monitored and taken without breaks can create the process of feedback inhibition, which can make you dependent on the hormone for the long term. There are excellent physicians out there who monitor the use of progesterone, but make sure you ask questions about follow up with saliva tests to assess the effects the cream is at the level of the tissue. Progesterone was actually the first contraceptive discovered, so too much of this can work against your fertility.

Here's an example of what I see in the clinic. I was seeing a patient who was using progesterone cream to help improve her progesterone levels because she was experiencing sore breasts consistently throughout the luteal phase, or second half, of her cycle and she wanted also to become pregnant. The cream helped for about ten months, then her symptoms began to return, and she started feeling out of balance emotionally. Saliva tests were conducted to measure her levels of progesterone, and these tests showed progesterone levels at 14,000. Normal for progesterone is 1,000 to 1,500! If not monitored closely, the use of hormone creams or any synthetic or bio-identical hormone replacement can result in a hormone imbalance.

Note: Your body is very intelligent, despite what you have been lead to believe when dealing with fertility issues, and is constantly trying to conserve energy while creating a balance overall. Taking a hormone is not the same as taking a vitamin. Whenever you take a hormone (any hormone) from outside the body on a consistent basis the body often slows down its own production of that hormone. The body is efficient. Why would it continue to make more hormone when it is getting the hormone from the medication you are taking. This process if you are taking the hormone for the long term can make you dependent on that hormone in some cases for life. This does not mean I think taking hormones such as thyroid hormone, for example, or hormones in cream form is bad and should be always avoided, based on what I have seen in the clinic many things can be done first before giving someone something they will have to take for the very long term. Keep in mind also that proper monitoring must be done to make sure you are at optimal levels.

If a hormone is low in someone who is in their twenties, thirties, forties, and fifties, it is usually low for a reason. The body is making it low due to feedback it is receiving or not receiving in the system. For example, if progesterone is low in a twenty-, thirty- or even forty- year old, it does not mean necessarily that the body is literally deficient, but instead, the reason progesterone is low could be the adrenals can be using up the progesterone due to a need to make more cortisol (the stress hormone), or the thyroid may not be making enough of a thyroid hormone called T3, which helps stimulate progesterone production. Both of these scenarios can result from stressors on the system.

Addressing the underlying cause is extremely important in addressing any hormone issue. Use of creams and other forms of hormone therapy can be used but in my opinion could be avoided in some women if steps to address thyroid and adrenal function occurred first. But if you choose to go down the hormone route, remember to make sure proper testing via saliva tests are done to ensure optimal levels of hormone acting on the organ tissues.

ESTROGEN DEFICIENCY

Low estrogen or estrogen deficiency affects the health of the eggs and therefore influences whether fertilization can take place. Gradual declining levels of estrogen normally occurs through perimenopause and menopause. Deficiency in estrogen can also occur when there is excessive stress on the system. One example of this is being underweight. The lack of body fat can negatively affect estrogen levels due to fat being one of the primary storage areas for estrogen.

Being underweight can disrupt the delicate balance of hormones by reducing the amount of gonadotrophin-releasing hormone (GnRH), which controls the secretion of follicle stimulating hormone (FSH) and luteinizing hormone (LH), all of which are important to a female's fertility. This can put stress on the system, which has been shown to impact a female's menstrual cycle and ovulation as discussed in chapter 9, step five, I Didn't Buy a Ticket for This Emotional Rollercoaster.

Depending on the type and amount of exercise a person does, for women who are underweight, excessive exercise can reduce the amount of fat in the body a bit too much. After a certain percentage of fat loss, the amount of sex hormones being produced can lower, and ovulation can be disrupted or the period even stops. Even a woman with regular cycles who is underweight is at risk of not producing the optimal balance of estrogen and progesterone to create and maintain a viable pregnancy.

Some women who are underweight say that this cannot be the reason they are not pregnant because they have been this weight all of their adult life. If there has not been a viable pregnancy while at that weight, it is possible that, though being underweight has not resulted in any disease process or disturbance in their cycle, it could be impacting fertility.

Being overweight can also contribute to low (or elevated) estrogen levels. In some women with polycystic ovaries or premature ovarian insufficiency who do not menstruate or menstruate very infrequently, their estrogen levels can be low (or elevated).

Whether weight is the issue causing low estrogen or not, when low levels of estrogen occur during reproductive years, this generally indicates that the egg may not become mature enough to contribute to a viable pregnancy or an egg may not be released at all. If estrogen remains low, then the brain may not receive a signal to release luteinizing hormone, the hormone that spikes when the egg is released.

Several factors can contribute to estrogen deficiency. Estrogen, like most of your reproductive hormones, is made from cholesterol, so your body needs a good supply of good cholesterol to optimize hormone production.

Studies have shown that some women with low HDL (protective cholesterol) levels can have low estrogen levels. Women who consume inadequate amounts of essential fatty acids (EFAs) in their diet encourage less than optimal estrogen production. Getting an abundance of EFA's not only encourages optimal estrogen production, it can actually improve part of your cholesterol picture, too.

HDLs, the good cholesterol, can increase when taking good fats. This happens by reducing liver enzyme activity that breaks down HDLs and could potentially protect against heart disease and possibly optimize their fertility. Step one, Develop a Fertile Eating Plan, and step three, Optimal Supplementation Program, discuss how to make sure you are getting clean healthy sources of EFAs in your system. Remember essential fatty acids are called essential because your body doesn't make them and they must come from our diet.

Factors that reduce availability of estrogen are as follows:

- Smoking (disrupts metabolism of estrogen and more of the inactive estrogen can be produced. This can result in estrogen dominance as well.)

- Low body weight (BMI 19 or less)
- Exercising too much (reduces levels of circulating estrogen)
- Insulin resistance (precursor to diabetes and present in many with PCOS)
- Any long-term physiological or emotional stress on the system

SYMPTOMS OF ESTROGEN DEFICIENCY

The following are some common symptoms of estrogen deficiency:

- Hot flashes
- Vaginal dryness
- Irregular periods
- Light periods
- Rapid skin aging
- Night sweats
- Excessive bone loss
- Amenorrhea: absence of the period

Remember, these symptoms can also be noted with other issues such as adrenal stress and thyroid issues, but your healthcare practitioner should consider and investigate estrogen deficiency if you are experiencing these symptoms. If estradiol is optimal or low, then looking at the thyroid and adrenals is the logical next step to address the symptoms listed.

If you are experiencing either estrogen dominance or estrogen deficiency, it is not all doom and gloom either. Herbs and some supplements have been shown to optimize estrogen levels in comparison to progesterone, which may improve fertility. Seeing an experienced herbalist, naturopath, or physician about this can get you started on a program to address less-than-optimal hormone fluctuation.

OTHER WEIGHT ISSUES

Overweight women and men (as well as men and women who are of normal weight) can experience a medical issue called insulin resistance. Insulin resistance most often occurs as a result of eating excess sugar, high glycemic carbohydrates, empty calories through sodas or soft drinks, excessive alcohol consumption, minimal amount of healthy protein, low amounts of good fat and high amounts of trans fat, and many times, lack of exercise. Sounds like the average American!!

Less frequently, the diet is not the issue and an underlying thyroid issue can cause a problem with the liver's ability to metabolize glucose (sugar). Insulin resistance can develop then develop as a result of a sluggish thyroid. Insulin resistance has also been correlated to the use of certain medications such as high blood pressure medications and difficulty metabolizing glucose (sugar) well has been associated with antidepressants.

It has been shown in many studies that insulin resistance is associated with inflammation in the body, which in turn can cause physiological stress and affect the output and regulation of estrogen, progesterone, and testosterone production. This can create estrogen dominance for females *and* males, estrogen deficiency in females and testosterone deficiency in males.

A woman who is overweight or underweight and has regular menstrual cycles may still have less than optimal balance of estrogen and progesterone. The best time in the cycle to test the estrogen/progesterone balance is seven days after ovulation. See chapter 3, "Determining Ovulation."

Seven days after ovulation, blood tests for FSH, estradiol, and progesterone can be performed. If a woman is experiencing estrogen dominance (i.e., too much estrogen with optimal progesterone, optimal estrogen with low progesterone, or excess estrogen and low progesterone), this can create an imbalance and impact fertility.

In men, too much estrogen compared to testosterone can cause estrogen dominance, leading to issues with fertility and potentially prostate health as well. When a male is under stress no matter what the cause (excess weight, emotional stress, chemical exposure, excessive alcohol or food sensitivities to name a few), it can cause testosterone to convert too quickly and too often into estrogen and lead to prostate issues, male fertility issues, low libido, and or increase in breast tissue. Saliva tests are a great way to assess whether this is happening in males.

Men can have blood tests for their hormones on any day since they don't have a cycle.

THYROID IMBALANCE: NORMAL IS NOT ALWAYS OPTIMAL

Studies have found that by the age of fifty, one in twelve women will have an issue with their thyroid. This increases to one in six by the age of sixty. According to the American Thyroid Association, women are five to eight times more susceptible to developing thyroid issues than men. But can thyroid issues for either sex impact your fertility?

The answer is yes! There is a critical relationship between the thyroid gland, the butterfly-shaped organ in your neck and nearly every aspect of fertility.

Think of the thyroid as the organ that either speeds up your body or slows it down. The thyroid helps you feel energetic but it also helps to slow you down to conserve energy. It is like your body's engine. In women, the thyroid can affect the ability to become pregnant and maintain a healthy pregnancy. It also affects postpartum health, successful breastfeeding, and even the health of your baby. In men common fertility issues such as low count can be attributed to issues with the thyroid, in part due to the thyroids relationship with testosterone.

Common fertility problems for females caused by both hypo- and hyperthyroidism are anovulation (i.e., no ovulation: an egg is not released or is not healthy enough to become fertilized or implant) and menstruation cycle irregularities.

Thyroid dysfunction can stop ovulation by upsetting the balance of the body's natural reproductive hormones. Elevated thyroid antibodies are also correlated with stillbirths, miscarriage, and even postnatal depression. Elevated antibodies have a strong correlation with less than optimal adrenal function.

A woman's ovaries and uterus need an optimal level of thyroid hormone in order to support reproduction. The thyroid helps to stimulate the production of progesterone and help the liver breakdown and metabolize estrogens in the body. Both of these processes help create the balance between estrogen and progesterone in women and testosterone and estrogen in men.

Even a subclinical or variation in thyroid levels can lead to issues with fertility. The American Society of Reproductive Medicine recommends treating women with Thyroid Stimulating Hormone (TSH) >4.0 if they are trying to conceive. TSH is the hormone that doctors typically monitor when looking at the thyroid. It comes from the brain and gives an indication of what the brain needs for thyroid hormone.

Some "normal ranges" can go up to 6.5 for TSH. Before IVF many doctors are recommending that TSH be less than 2.5. So as you can see, some medical doctors and researchers are saying that "normal" TSH levels aren't good enough for some women to increase their chances of creating a pregnancy.

From a holistic perspective, we have discussed what estrogen dominance (either excess estrogen or low progesterone in women and excess estrogen compared to testosterone in men) means.

When a women experiences excess estrogen in the system, this can result in an increase in the amount of thyroid binding globulin (TBG) circulating in the body. TBG is a protein that attaches to freely circulating thyroid hormone and converts it into bound thyroid hormone, which is not usable. This protein is carrying the thyroid hormone somewhere but while the hormone is bound to TBG it can't be used. An example might be a bottle of wine. In this analogy you can't see through the bottle. Remember I recommended LIMIT alcohol consumption to no more than 3-4 drinks per week. ☺ Okay back to the example, the wine is T4, and a cap on the wine is TBG. As long as that cap (TBG) is attached securely to that bottle of wine the wine (thyroid hormone T4) can't be used. But when you disconnect the cap from the bottle the wine can be used. Excessive estrogen increases the TBG and decreases the effectiveness of the thyroid hormone.

Therefore even if your blood tests show your thyroid levels to be normal, you may have less active thyroid hormone than you think if you TBG is high. This commonly happens to women on the oral contraceptive pill. If the extra estrogen in their system from the pill causes TBG to increase they can experience less active thyroid hormone in their system and develop a sluggish thyroid. Typical symptoms seen with a sluggish thyroid are as follows:

➤ Weight gain
➤ Difficulty losing weight
➤ Constipation
➤ Depression
➤ Fatigue
➤ Dry skin
➤ Irregular menstrual cycle
➤ No menstrual cycle
➤ Hormonal imbalances
➤ Low libido
➤ Anxiety
➤ High blood pressure
➤ Elevated cholesterol
➤ Diabetes
➤ Some autoimmune issues (Hashimoto's disease)

Even women or men of normal weight can have a sluggish thyroid if they experience any of the above symptoms.

Mia came to me after having difficulty conceiving her second child. She was lean, and all of her life, she did not have to watch what she ate. She had issues with progesterone, which we were working on. I saw Mia early in my career, and because she was lean and had no weight issue, I wasn't concerned about her thyroid. After six months on the program, Mia wasn't pregnant, so I began to think that possibly her thyroid was overactive, that is, working too hard. I was shocked when the hormone levels came back and showed her thyroid levels to be in the very low range, indicating that her thyroid was actually sluggish not overactive. Since one of the thyroid hormones T3 (which comes from T4) helps to make progesterone, we created a program to support the conversion of T4 to T3 and then the body was able to use more T3 to stimulate the ovaries to make additional progesterone. Therefore by following the Five-Step Fertility Solution™, Mia was able to optimize her progesterone production and she noted improved thickness of her endometrial lining. Mia noted her periods had improved, as well; they felt like they did back when she was in her twenties.

The thyroid is extremely important not only in helping to create a pregnancy but also maintaining one. Women with a sluggish thyroid (hypothyroidism) need to produce 40 percent more thyroid hormone during pregnancy because the baby relies on this hormone from the mother for its growth and development. For that reason, many doctors monitor and increase a woman's thyroid hormone dosage when they become pregnant, and evaluate the level throughout the pregnancy for necessary adjustments. But unfortunately if a woman doesn't already have a thyroid issue, the thyroid is rarely monitored in pregnancy even though the stress and demands of pregnancy can impact thyroid health.

Janice came to me to work toward creating a pregnancy. After six months, she was pregnant and happy as could be. But at nineteen weeks, she came back to me concerned that the growth of the baby had slowed, and the doctors weren't sure if the baby was going to make it. They told Janice to give it a few more weeks and "see what happens." But Janice didn't feel right about it and came to discuss it with me. Janice did not have a thyroid issue by medical standards prior to pregnancy, and therefore the doctors didn't evaluate her thyroid function during pregnancy.

I showed her studies of sluggish fetal growth related to less than optimal thyroid function during pregnancy. So she went back to her physician and had her thyroid tested. Thankfully, we had tests that doctor had done prior to pregnancy. When we compared them, we could see her thyroid hormones had changed dramatically. Though they were still in the normal range, they were teetering on the edge of being abnormal. Armed with the studies to show her doctor that a thyroid issue was related to poor fetal growth rates and increased mortality rates, the doctor decided to treat her thyroid. Thankfully, the fetus growth improved, and Janice delivered a healthy baby girl at full term.

ELEVATED PROLACTIN

A sluggish thyroid that impacts your fertility can also be correlated with an increase in the secretion of prolactin, the hormone that induces and maintains the production of breast milk in a postpartum woman.

However, elevated prolactin can happen in women who are not pregnant. When this happens, the elevated prolactin can sometimes suppress estrogen, which could prevent ovulation, causing irregular or absent monthly cycles. There are situations however when prolactin is elevated but estrogen is normal and oftentimes this can be related to thyroid issues.

Elevated prolactin can sometimes be overlooked when there are no other symptoms associated with the high levels. Some women with elevated prolactin will experience discharge from the nipple that is either clear or milky. If this is observed discharge from a woman's breast should be investigated by her doctor. When the doctor clears any serious health issues related to the breast discharge, the thyroid should be checked as well.

Prolactin is a stress-dependent hormone. One theory of how prolactin is related to hypothyroidism is that elevated prolactin increases a hormone that increases the release of TSH. Another theory is related to stress. When stress is high, this can stimulate the production of cortisol and in many increased cortisol can decrease prolactin, but in some, such as women with endometriosis increased cortisol and increased prolactin have been found. With increase stress the conversion of T4 to T3 (the more active thyroid hormone) slows down. This can lead to less than optimal levels of active T3 circulating in the system and potentially decreased reproductive hormones such as progesterone. Therefore, whenever prolactin is elevated (unless prolactin is supposed to be elevated such as in a woman who is breastfeeding) the thyroid should be fully assessed.

Treatment for elevated prolactin, especially if a pituitary tumor is involved, is usually a drug called Dostinex or a dopamine agonist. This medication does lower prolactin levels effectively but does not address why prolactin was elevated in the first place. Long-term use of these types of medications, however, can be associated with lowered progesterone levels. If you are taking Dostinex or a similar drug to lower prolactin levels, it is important to discuss the potential effects this can have on your fertility and what other alternatives you may have. There can be an increase in pregnancies in women who have just started taking Dostinex or similar drugs for elevated prolactin but after a few months (3-6) if no pregnancy has occurred there is often an underlying issue still needing to be addressed.

In my opinion, if all serious complications have been ruled out for someone who has elevated prolactin, it may be more effective for her fertility to address the underlying cause of the elevated prolactin than to just try to suppress it because its elevation is a sign that the body is out of balance and possibly that the thyroid is in need of evaluation and support.

OVERACTIVE THYROID

Less commonly seen, but still significant, is the overactive thyroid. An overactive thyroid can be producing too much hormone, therefore, speeding up processes such as heart rate and hormone metabolism. For example, typically with an overactive thyroid, cholesterol goes down quickly due to the liver speeding up its metabolism of cholesterol, while with an underactive thyroid, the liver becomes sluggish and cholesterol can rise. Typical symptoms of overactive thyroid are as follows:

➢ Irritability
➢ Sweats
➢ Heart palpitations
➢ Loose bowels
➢ Bulging eyes
➢ Excessive weight loss for no reason
➢ Anxiety
➢ Racing pulse

To complicate matters, you may experience a combination of these symptoms when the thyroid is either over or underactive, so assessing the state of thyroid output through blood tests is helpful.

The bottom line is when you are dealing with fertility issues, a full assessment of your thyroid should be done in order to rule out less than optimal thyroid output, an overactive thyroid, or elevated thyroid antibodies.

THYROID ANTIBODIES

What are thyroid antibodies? Antibodies are created due to a signal from the immune-system. For example, antibodies are created in our body to neutralize foreign invaders such as viruses and bacteria. This is a welcome reaction to keep us healthy. However other antibodies can over time cause significant health issues if not decreased significantly. One example is when thyroid antibodies are created by our immune system to attack the thyroid gland, to slow it down, usually as a result of stress on the system.

Why would the body turn on itself and attack its own organ tissue? It seems as if the body has gone haywire, but in fact, this can be an intelligent way that organ systems communicate with each other.

When the adrenals have been taxed for long periods of time and the physiologic gas tank (the adrenals) is getting empty, *both* cortisol and DHEA are low, which occurs in some people with long-term chronic stress. When this happens, the adrenals may communicate with the immune system to look for ways to slow the body down in order to conserve more energy. Since the thyroid is one of the most important organs to regulate metabolism and energy levels, by slowing this organ system down and decreasing absorption of nutrients such as iron, it can allow the individual to feel sluggish and tired, which can result in expending less energy overall. Great for the body to conserve energy but not great for the person who is tired, exhausted and feeling terrible.

If the individual addresses the sources of the stress, finds a better balance, and rejuvenates the adrenal glands, the thyroid antibodies often go down and thyroid function, as well as adrenal function, improves. This allows fertility to be optimized in some individuals. Remember, though, this stress is not always emotional and very often is related to some physiological stress on the system, like what was experienced by Nancy and Al.

Nancy and Al had been trying to become pregnant for six to seven years. Nothing was happening, and they were at their wits' end. After coming to the clinic, I suggested testing the thyroid and the adrenals. Both Nancy and Al assured me that these systems must have been tested because they were told there were no other tests that could be performed. Their situation was simply unexplained.

They gathered their previous info for me to review. I noted that only thyroid stimulating hormone (TSH) had been tested for the thyroid and no adrenal hormones had been tested in the information provided to me.

Nancy and Al went back to their GP to get their thyroid tested, TSH, FT4, FT3, thyroid antibodies, reverse T3, and two adrenal hormones tested cortisol (done in the a.m.) and DHEA.

The most significant findings were that Nancy's thyroid antibodies, specifically anti-thyroglobulin and thyroid peroxidase antibodies were 8,700 and 5,500, respectively. Normal levels for these hormones is less than thirty.

Thyroid antibodies had not been tested before because TSH was normal and, according to Dr. Mark Starr (author of Type 2 Hypothyroidism), physicians learn in medical school that if TSH is normal, then the thyroid is fine and antibodies do not need to be tested.

However, if you ask most physicians what will eventually happen to the thyroid when thyroid antibodies are elevated, even if TSH is normal, most will say that the thyroid will eventually fail. But as long as TSH is normal (according to Dr. Starr), most physicians won't do anything about thyroid health at that time. They simply wait for the thyroid to fail and then begin treatment.

This approach can be detrimental to your fertility. A 2008 review of studies show elevated thyroid antibodies (even when TSH is normal) to be associated with increased miscarriage rate and infertility. Elevated thyroid antibodies have also been associated with issues such as celiac disease or gluten sensitivity, which can impact fertility. Oftentimes, polycystic ovaries and thyroid antibodies are associated.

Therefore, it is important to address the probable stressors that contributed to the adrenals being wiped out and potentially triggering an immune system response to attack the thyroid and slow it down to conserve energy.

For Nancy, I recommended she remove gluten and dairy from her diet. Her antibodies came down to 7,500 and 3,000 respectively. I also talked about work-life balance and avoiding exposure to chemicals. Nancy had worked for many years in a printing factory where chemicals and fumes were abundant. This is where her trouble with thyroid and adrenal health may have begun due to the negative effects that chemical exposure can have on thyroid function and overall stress on the system.

About 30 percent of our patients end up needing thyroid medications such as Thyroxine, combo of T4/T3, or natural thyroid extract from their doctor to help with the antibodies. Many require extra support of the adrenal glands, but this is not usually handled medically unless the patient is diagnosed with Addison's disease (too little adrenal hormone) or Cushing's disease (excessive adrenal hormone). Many do extremely well on the Five-Step Fertility Solution™ and become pregnant. Thankfully Nancy saw an open-minded physician who put her on a combination of T4 and T3 based on the studies relating thyroid antibodies to fertility issues and miscarriage. I continued to work to support her adrenal glands and added the nutrients selenium and inositol since these have been shown to be correlated with lowering thyroid antibodies.

The antibody levels continued to come down over another three to four months, then Nancy called me to say she was pregnant. She went on to have another viable pregnancy only ten months after her first child was born. "It took us almost seven years to create our daughter, and I was sure it would take at least two years or so for the second one," she said. "But the program worked like a charm." For Nancy, once the thyroid and adrenals were moving toward balance, her reproductive function followed along.

In recent years the nutrients selenium and myo inositol have been shown in studies to be effective at reducing thyroid antibodies as well. As discussed in the chapter titled "What's Supp?," a broad-spectrum multivitamin is important to have as a prenatal supplement for men and women but when thyroid antibodies are present making sure selenium is taken in adequate amounts (up to 150–200 mcg total selenium for all sources) along with myo-inositol (1.5 to 4 g depending on your diagnosis) can be beneficial in addressing the antibody issue. Nutritional supplements to address a specific health-care need should always be considered and monitored by a qualified healthcare professional.

HOW DOES THE THYROID WORK?

Based on everything discussed in the last few sections you may have some idea of what hormones the thyroid produces. In this section I am going to attempt to pull it all together to help further your understanding about the significance of thyroid function and its hormonal actions on our overall health.

The following is a list of its activities in our body:

➢ Carbohydrate, protein, and fat metabolism
➢ Vitamin utilization
➢ Energy production
➢ Digestive processes
➢ Muscle and nerve activity
➢ Hormone secretion
➢ Sexual and reproductive health
➢ Cardiovascular function
➢ Metabolism of cholesterol
➢ Helps to regulate blood pressure

The production and release of thyroid hormones are normally thought to be controlled by thyroid stimulating hormone (TSH), which is secreted by the pituitary gland. In fact, as discussed, this is the gold standard test when physicians look at the thyroid. However, it appears that TSH really only tells us what the brain needs for thyroid hormone and not what the rest of the body needs. We have found this to be true when TSH is normal but classic thyroid symptoms persist and actual thyroid hormone output is low compared to the optimal ranges gathered over the years.

The thyroid gland produces the thyroid hormones T4, T3, T2, T1, and T0. T1 and T2 have often been ignored and considered unimportant by most of the medical professionals because in the past they haven't been sure of their importance. T4 is given the most attention, but some doctors are now paying attention to T3, which is crucial for thyroid health, as well.

T4 is the main thyroid hormone. It contains four iodine bonds that we want to convert into T3 when enough selenium, zinc, chromium, iron and iodine are present. This happens in the thyroid but also in the liver, the gut, skeletal muscles and brain. If these nutrients aren't present at optimal levels in the body or if the body is under significant stress, the larger portion of T3 could end up being inactive and nonfunctioning. This is important because active T3 helps to stimulate progesterone and testosterone production, which in turn influences estrogen. The importance of assessing the amounts and balance of these hormones in trying to conceive is paramount.

If your doctor has looked at TSH and says your thyroid is fine but you still haven't created a viable pregnancy, it is very important for you to have the thyroid fully checked out and make sure the results are optimal, not just normal. Practitioners trained in my Fertility Mentoring Program through the Baby Maker Network are very familiar with our optimal ranges.

There is also a test that can help you determine if your T3 levels are active or mostly inactive. You could have normal T4 levels and a normal TSH but if T3 is low or there is too much inactive T3 then despite "normal" values, the effect of the hormones are less than optimal. Poor conversion of T4 to T3 that results in too much Reverse T3 (the inactive form of T3) can be related to inadequate progesterone and testosterone. Reverse T3 is a great test to help determine the quality of T3 being produced.

Urinary iodine tests are also very important. In some parts of the United States, Australia, and Europe, iodine is showing up as low in adults and children, despite the increased use of iodized salts (salt with iodine). This is likely because there is an ingredient in iodized salts called chloride that can block the absorption of iodine into your system, and the amount of iodine in the iodized salts then is not sufficient. Or it could also result from people not using salt at all because they were told salt is bad for them. In addition if they have a poor diet that contains processed foods and drinks that contain chemicals that block iodine such as energy drinks; low iodine levels can be a significant issue.

Less than optimal iodine for mothers who are pregnant can lead to significant health and intellectual issues for her children and either issues during pregnancy or postpartum.

The most common question that is asked when the thyroid is discussed or when a less than optimal level of thyroid hormone is identified is "Why didn't my doctor tell me this?"

My only answer is that your doctor may only go by what he or she learned in medical school when they discussed TSH and may not be reading updated research.

Take Juliette, for example. Sue was told her thyroid was fine. She experienced fertility issues for five years. Several IVF attempts never resulted in a pregnancy, and she reported to me that she had a short luteal phase.

Her TSH levels were 3.5, perfectly normal according to her doctor. When her free T4 and free T3 levels were tested, her T4 looked great but T3 was low. This often means T4 is not converting well into T3. This is relevant because T3 needs to be active and created in adequate amounts to stimulate progesterone. She was scheduled to have her next IVF attempt in five months. Her supplementation program was assessed, and she was given nutritionals and herbs to support her thyroid. After six weeks, she was tested again, and her Free T3 levels started to improve and her luteal phase started to lengthen, which often correlates with improved progesterone production.

At the fifth-month mark, her luteal phase was a normal fourteen days, and she decided she was comfortable with beginning her IVF cycle the cycle after next, but she didn't have to. She became pregnant the cycle before she was meant to start IVF. This couple and so many that I see had no prior pregnancies either naturally or with IVF until after she worked on optimizing her thyroid health.

HERBS TO SUPPORT THYROID HEALTH
There are some wonderful herbs to support thyroid health that we tend to use frequently:

- Withania somnifera: an Ayurvedic herb, has been shown to be supportive of thyroid health by optimizing T4 levels.
- Bacopa Monnieri: a Chinese herb, has been shown to be correlated with increasing T4 levels, as well.
- Bladderwrack or Fucus Vesiculosus: a seaweed that for some can be supportive for the thyroid to add iodine in the system. Too much iodine could cause problems though, especially if thyroid antibodies are present. Before starting any iodine make sure thyroid antibodies are tested and not elevated. Then discuss the best dose to start with to help support iodine levels in the body.

BUT MY DOCTOR SAYS MY THYROID IS FINE!
Frequently, patients tell me that their doctor has tested their thyroid hormone levels and told them their thyroid levels are within normal

parameters. However, when I see them, they are presenting with symptoms of either hypo- or hyperthyroidism. This is frustrating for these patients as the symptoms of a subclinical thyroid issue are numerous and impact their general wellbeing. Unfortunately, you can still have the symptoms of illnesses long before they are picked up in blood tests. This is due to many factors, some of which are discussed in Dr. Mark Starr's excellent resource book entitled *Type 2 Hypothyroidism.* If you suspect you may have a sluggish thyroid, this book is a great resource and has some good information that you can share with your physician.

The following tests are also helpful:

- FT4
- FT3
- Reverse T3
- Thyroid antibodies
- Urinary iodine levels

In addition, it can be helpful to chart your temperature during your cycle. Low temperatures, below 36.0 Celsius or below 96.8 Fahrenheit, first thing in the morning before you get out of bed (when taken with an oral digital thermometer) could signify suboptimal thyroid function. An inefficient rise in temperature after ovulation may mean sluggish progesterone, which could be related to the thyroid. In men, basal body temperatures taken with an oral digital thermometer below 36.1 Celsius or 97 degrees Fahrenheit can indicate low thyroid function. One temperature however doesn't say much. Look at a series of temperatures throughout your cycle, or for men for at least 5-10 days.

I AM ALREADY ON THYROID MEDICATION. HOW DO I KNOW IF IT'S WORKING?
If you are currently on medication for thyroid issues but still dealing with fertility issues, then it is time to get your medication reassessed.

TSH may be normal and your doctor says everything is fine but this is only assessing part of the story. Some patients who are on T4 (thyroxine) to support their thyroid can become Thyroxine resistant.

Take Helen, for instance. Helen and her husband had been trying to conceive for three years. Helen had been on thyroid medication for six years.

She was taking Thyroxine, which is T4 only, the main hormone your thyroid produces from iodine. Her temperatures remained low despite improvement in her symptoms, and her overall health was up and down.

Helen went to a forward-thinking doctor, who explained that even though her TSH levels were normal while she was on Thyroxine, it doesn't mean her thyroid was working optimally. He tested reverse T3, a test to indicate if there is too much inactive T3 in the system in comparison to active T3. Finding that reverse T3 was elevated, he changed Helen's thyroid medication to natural thyroid extract. Not everyone does well on thyroid extract also called Armor Thyroid but it agreed with Helen. Her reverse T3 came down to normal, and a pregnancy resulted eight months later while following the Five-Step Fertility Solution.

It is never a good idea to self-medicate, change your medications, or stop your medications. Always seek the advice of a physician. A great resource for open-minded thyroid doctors around the world is http://www.thyroid-info.com/topdrs/.

Some of my patients reading about Helen's story have wanted to switch to natural thyroid extract but this isn't always the best decision for everyone. I have had women taking natural thyroid extract who were doing well at first but overtime I noticed an issue with their T4 levels. T4 was decreasing steadily over time, which can create other issues. In some women, low T4 can cause their once regular cycles to become irregular or stop all together. Thankfully this doesn't happen with everyone who takes natural thyroid extract prescribed by their doctor. But it emphasizes the importance of monitoring all thyroid levels closely once on a medication to see if it is the right medication for you.

Other patients have done extremely well on a combination of T4 and T3 in one medication. While others just needed the additional nutrients such as iodine, selenium, zinc, chromium, and iron to keep their thyroid working optimally.

I hope this helps you realize that finding a person who understands thyroid function and what options are out there to address it is extremely important.

THYROID MEDICATIONS IN PREGNANCY

While we are discussing thyroid medications, let's talk about other thyroid medications which is essentially hormone replacement, i.e. it is giving hormones to the body to replace hormones the body isn't making in large enough and quantities to be effective. Some doctors are hesitant to recommend thyroid medications during pregnancy due to some older research studies speculating that these medications were associated with miscarriages, could affect a baby's growth in the womb, result in a less than full-term pregnancy, and even cause birth defects. This can be an old outdated approach.

Mary's doctor diagnosed her with hypothyroidism shortly after she and her husband, Mark, were married. The medication came with instructions, as well as the precautionary warning that women should not become pregnant while taking the medication because it could cause miscarriages, fetal complications, and prevent them from carrying a child full-term. Thankfully this warning has been removed from many of the precautionary warnings.

Every year, Mary returned to her doctor to continue her thyroid prescription. After seven years, Mary and Mark, now in their early forties had accepted the fact that they wouldn't have children because Mary was on thyroid medication. At an annual checkup, Mary's gynecologist inquired whether the couple was planning to have children. Mary explained that they couldn't become pregnant because she was on thyroid medication. Her doctor referenced her medication and the dosage and stated that the dosage she was on wasn't high enough to have any negative impact on the baby she may carry or increase her risk of miscarriage. In their early forties, if Mary and Mark were interested in becoming pregnant, they still had time. After discussing this change of events, the couple decided this was their opportunity to attempt to become pregnant. After believing pregnancy was not an option for them for so many years, they became pregnant in only two months of timed intercourse whereas before they were avoiding intercourse at ovulation due to the fear that they would miscarry or have a child with severe birth defects.

Mary's experience is one reason why it is important to talk to your medical professional and fertility team. Per the outdated warnings associated with thyroid medication at the dose she was taking, Mary's previous physician had advised her not to become pregnant. Her gynecologist, however, was more experienced with thyroid disorders and their effect on pregnancy. Unfortunately, Mary would have never known that she could conceive and carry a child if her gynecologist hadn't inquired about it. In this couple's case, the warning that came with Mary's medication wasn't relevant to her dosage.

ADRENAL FATIGUE AND ADRENAL EXHAUSTION

Another area commonly overlooked when dealing with fertility issues is adrenal hormone output and its impact on fertility.

Let's first discuss normal adrenal function.

The adrenals are small organs that sit on top of the kidneys. They might be tiny, but they play a huge role in overall health and your fertility.

The inside of the adrenal gland, called the medulla, produces hormones such as cortisol and adrenaline. These hormones help us combat stress from outside and inside of our body.

The outer portion of the adrenals, the cortex, produce hormones such as estrogen and progesterone in small amounts, hormones that help regulate blood pressure and blood sugar levels, and hormones that impact growth and development.

If we focus on the inner portion of the adrenals, the medulla and its response to stress, this is where the fight or flight mechanism comes into play. The fight or flight response is a natural response in all of us and occurs when our body and mind either unconsciously or consciously perceives danger. Hundreds of years ago, if a person was stalked by a wild animal (for instance, a lion), the fight or flight response would be activated and they would to fight the lion or flee. During this instance of perceived danger, a stress response occurs, you either grab your spear and attack or you run away.

During this response, stress hormones are released into the system by the adrenals to prepare the body to fight or flee. This hormonal response sets off alarm bells in the rest of the body and the body reacts to the stress. When the stimulatory stress hormones are released, our digestion can slow down, our immune system drops, the reproductive system can be shut off. All of those systems use up a lot of energy so during a stress response if we are being chased like a lion, some systems slow down to allow more energy to be directed to the task at hand which is defending yourself or getting the heck out of dodge.

Other physiological changes occur. Increased blood flow is directed toward the muscles. The heartbeat increases. The body begins to sweat to release excess heat created in the process, and brain activity changes, decreasing activity in the logical thinking centers of the brain and increasing activity to the more reactive part of the brain so a person can respond quickly.

After the perceived stress is gone, that is, the person defeated the lion in battle or ran up a tree to escape, over time the body can rebalance itself. The function of the digestive system, immune system, brain, heart, circulation, and so on can return to normal within a period of time.

This is a much needed response to help us cope and survive, but in today's world, the adrenals can become overloaded. People no longer typically have wild animals to contend with, but instead, there are constant deadlines, relationships to manage, stress at work or stress because a person is out of work, financial issues, health issues including fertility issues, and family issues to deal with on a daily basis.

Those dealing with fertility issues have the additional stress of doctor appointments to manage, blood to be drawn, ultrasounds to be performed, medications to be taken, procedures scheduled and performed, pregnancy and ovulation tests to take, and temperatures to keep track of, as well as the stress related to not knowing what is going to happen month after month.

Therefore, when these stressors are consistent and chronic, there may not be a lion chasing the person dealing with fertility issues, but the chronic stress over time can impact reproductive hormone function. For example, when cortisol is called upon to be produced due to consistent stress over a long period of time, and there is little time for the body to rebalance itself, the body can utilize the hormone progesterone to make more cortisol. It has also been shown in some studies that elevated cortisol levels can be correlated with low testosterone production as well.

Stress can, therefore, initially cause an increase in cortisol levels that may correlate with lower testosterone levels (which can subsequently lead to an issue with estrogen levels, as well, because estrogen comes from testosterone) and lower progesterone levels. In addition, chronic stress over a period of years can eventually cause the body to decrease cortisol output because it is unable to keep up with the demands. Everything ends up slowing down at that point, including production of important reproductive hormones.

Steve and Emily were just nonstop. They had been trying for a baby for over four years and had fourteen procedures including IUI, and fresh and frozen IVF cycles. When I saw them, they were at their wits' end. Both walked into my office and literally fell into the chairs, each with a coffee in hand. As I looked at them with their glaringly obvious dark circles below their eyes, Emily began to tell their story.

Two weeks before, they had their last frozen embryo attempt, and none of the embryos had thawed. Emily began to cry. Immediately, Steve perked up and finished by telling me their fertility history. Clearly trying to be strong for Emily, Steve would periodically reach over and hold Emily's hand or gently stroke her back as she wept and attempted to answer my questions.

Through the consultation, I asked whether they had any other stressors they were dealing with over the last few years. They both looked at each other. Like any couple in their late thirties, they had their fair share of stress. They had renovated their house, moved twice, and sold an investment property to help pay expenses. One parent had died, and work stress was consistent for them both. Their exhaustion developed over time.

The more difficulty they had, the harder they worked. Using their work as a distraction and sometimes alcohol as a stress management tool, their communication waned, and their relationship was beginning to suffer. Emily wanted to do another cycle right away, but Steve who was worried about Emily's mental health and their financial health had had enough. He wanted them to take time out to get their health and life back and if necessary, face the fact that they may never have a child so they could get on with life.

I explained that the adrenal glands are like a gas tank, and the adrenal hormones are similar to gas in the gas tank. The thyroid gland is like the engine of a car. I explained that I felt they were both out of gas (low adrenal function) and their engines (thyroid) was probably sluggish as well.

Saliva tests looking at cortisol levels throughout the day confirmed that the cortisol from the adrenals was not peaking in the morning when it should and for Emily it was rising before bed when it should be its lowest, which affected her ability to fall asleep. Blood tests confirmed that free testosterone was low for Steve, and progesterone was low for Emily.

Note: Naturopaths and some doctors often use saliva tests to determine adrenal function because it is best to test the stress hormone cortisol throughout the day. Instead of having blood drawn 4 times a day to monitor the normal fluctuation of cortisol, filling up 4 tubes with saliva at work, at home or wherever you may be is much more convenient. Testing saliva gives an indication of which hormones are already absorbed and acting on the tissues, not just those that have been floating around in the blood. In addition, the stress related to having a blood test, due to either perceived stress of having the blood drawn or the actual poking of the needle into the skin, can cause the body to respond and increase cortisol as a response to that stress and may not give a good resting level of cortisol through the day.

Cortisol, a stimulatory hormone, has a typical pattern throughout the day. It should be highest in the morning so you can wake up and have energy to start the day and gradually decreases through the day. It is lowest at night to help us fall asleep and stay asleep.

Like many of my patients, Emily and Steve wanted the herbs from the program to fix them, but after three months on the herbs without feeling better (due to avoiding following steps four and five of the five steps in the Five-Step Fertility Solution™), both Steve and Emily were getting frustrated and were ready to give up.

At our next consultation, I asked them both, "Do you have room for a baby in your lives?" I directed my next question to Emily. "Do you honestly think that with the way you are feeling right now, you would feel well during pregnancy and then be able to care for a newborn while breastfeeding and trying to manage working as well?"

Tears began to well up in her eyes again, and though she didn't respond verbally, she looked down and her head slowly shook back and forth.

"Isn't it time you both started to take responsibility for your health and wellbeing and stop looking at something outside of you to be the only thing to make you stronger, healthier, and eventually more fertile?" I asked. As you can imagine, silence filled the consult room.

I didn't see Steve and Emily for six months. They had canceled their next appointment and had not returned our phone calls until one day when Emily called to reschedule. The couple that I saw walk through the door at their next appointment was significantly different from the two people who had dragged themselves into the clinic coffee in hand months earlier.

"How have you been?" I asked.

This time Emily answered, no tears and only a shade of the dark circles under her eyes that I had seen before, "We took your comments to heart last time we saw you and made some changes in our lives," she said. "I got a new job, working full-time but with less stress, and full-time at this job is actually less hours than what I was doing. Steve is working at the same place but has stopped working late so we can both do some sort of activity or exercise most days after work. Weekends are for relaxing, and we don't try to cram our weekends full anymore and, when needed, take time for ourselves."

It seemed like I was speaking to a different couple.

When retested, their hormone levels had improved but were still not optimal, so we started the process again. Steve and Emily had begun to make the changes to their eating plan as well and were feeling better for it. They used some of their vacation hours from work to go away for two weeks and were planning another shorter trip in a few months. They continued their supplementation program, as previously discussed, and restarted the herbs. Finally, they were starting to feel stronger and more resilient.

They decided to spend the following six months preparing themselves for IVF. Unfortunately, the following IVF cycle didn't create a viable pregnancy. However, this time while Emily and Steve felt sad and disappointed, their resilience prevailed, and they decided to take a break from all the tests and appointments while continuing to implement all they learned in the program including the herbs. I said I would recommend an appointment in three months' time since they were in the maintenance phase of the program. It wasn't a very long break, however, because the second menstrual cycle after IVF, Emily called to let us know she was pregnant naturally for the first time in her life.

HERBS TO SUPPORT ADRENAL HEALTH

When the adrenals are involved, it can take some time for them to recover and improve fertility overall. Stress management is a massive step in the right direction but can be helped along and recovery time shortened by the appropriate use of herbs called adaptogens. These are herbs that help the body adapt to stress and exert a normalizing effect on adrenal function.

Withania Somnifera, also discussed with the thyroid, can be used to support adrenal health as well.

Rehmannia glutinosa, a Chinese herb, is excellent for helping balance adrenal health when stress has been chronic, that is, long term.

Licorice is a Chinese herb that is also common in balancing adrenal function. Higher potency has been associated with increasing blood pressure, so (as with all herbs above) consulting a professional herbalist, naturopath, or physician familiar with herb drug interactions is important.

Rhodiola rosea (also known as golden root) can be an effective herb for restoration of the adrenal glands. Studies have shown rhodiola to be effective against fatigue, which is often associated with adrenal fatigue and exhaustion.

Siberian ginseng and Panax or Korean ginseng have also been related to supporting adrenal function.

It is always important to see a practitioner who is experienced in dispensing herbs before beginning an herbal protocol. It is important that an individualized formulation be put together for your particular situation.

TESTS TO ASSESS ADRENAL FUNCTION

CORTISOL

As discussed, blood tests for cortisol can be done but may not be as revealing as saliva tests where you can take samples throughout the day. Saliva tests for adrenal function can be ordered online in the United States from a company called Canary Club. Their website is canaryclub.org. In Australia Clinical Labs and Path Labs are often used for saliva testing and require a referral from a practitioner. Look for the adrenal hormone profile. Always have an experienced health-care practitioner help you assess these results.

DHEA

Dehydroepiandrosterone (DHEA) is also another hormone secreted by the adrenals. When the body is managing stressors well, DHEA and cortisol levels are quite balanced. However, when the body experiences stress, oftentimes when cortisol rises, DHEA falls. When the flight or fight response is over, and the body is able to recover, DHEA returns to normal, along with cortisol.

In the short term, if stress is persistent, whether this be physiological stress only (cold, flu, infection, eating gluten when sensitive or intolerant) or physiological stress as a result of emotional stress, cortisol can remain high and DHEA low for longer periods. Since DHEA is often referred to as the anti-aging hormone, lower levels of DHEA could be associated with faster cellular degeneration or cells that are aging faster. This would also be true even more so with chronic stress when both DHEA and cortisol become low and your physiologic gas tank is almost empty.

Some doctors have utilized DHEA to support egg health in women doing IVF if they are older than thirty-eight or not responding well to IVF medication. DHEA at times is administered in these women without testing DHEA in blood or saliva as part of an IVF protocol. This can result in women taking this hormone who do not need it; therefore, many will experience increased side effects of DHEA like hair falling out, acne, and aggression in some women. The other consequence of DHEA supplementation if not monitored appropriately is a hormone imbalance between testosterone and estrogen. DHEA is a precursor to testosterone, and when supplementing with DHEA (which is a hormone), testosterone levels can rise to abnormal amounts for women. This can result in increasing estrogen levels as well. If bad estrogen increases as a result then this could be detrimental to a woman's health. Careful monitoring of DHEA, estradiol levels and estrone levels should be done via saliva tests when DHEA is given orally.

Women are often told that 7-keto DHEA will not cause an imbalance because it does not convert to testosterone, but based on clinical data, especially with saliva testing, even 7-keto DHEA can convert into testosterone and contribute to a hormonal imbalance. The confusion may be due to most physicians utilizing blood tests to check DHEA versus saliva tests or not testing DHEA prior to administering it. Remember, blood tests do not reflect what is actually going on at the level of the tissues, only what hormone is circulating in the blood with the potential to act on the tissues.

Take Sue, for example. She was forty-seven years old and trying to become pregnant for nearly twelve years. I saw her in the clinic, and, as one could imagine, she was very frustrated. During a few conversations, Sue would become rather angry and agitated, and she felt as though these symptoms were progressing beyond her control. She had reported to me that she had been taking 7-keto DHEA for the last eighteen months and on and off previously during her years of IVF. Although her doctor tested DHEA in her blood over this period of time, testosterone was never tested. DHEA always did look to be normal in the blood, but due to Sue's continued agitation and anger and long-term use of DHEA, I decided to test via saliva tests. The results came back showing Sue had normal DHEA levels in the saliva, but her testosterone was 1,500 (normal levels of testosterone in the saliva are between fifteen and ninety).

Due to the way that DHEA and cortisol are balanced, if a person is low in DHEA, they are not likely deficient unless they are over sixty-five years of age, but instead there is an imbalance due to stress. Supplementing with DHEA in these people without addressing the stress through effective stress management may only end up increasing testosterone levels and creating a hormonal imbalance. Most people in their thirties and forties are not going to be truly deficient in DHEA, like someone in their seventies. Instead, less than optimal balance of cortisol and DHEA normally occurs at any earlier age due to stress. Therefore, addressing what is causing the stress and following the Five-Step Fertility Solution™ can help to rebalance the adrenal hormones and optimize fertility.

If DHEA treatment is being considered, a full adrenal and testosterone profile should be checked via blood and saliva. If DHEA is administered, the levels of DHEA, testosterone, and estrogen should be monitored in both blood and saliva. Based on clinical studies with patients taking DHEA who became pregnant, most pregnancies appeared to happen in the short term, that is, a few months after administering the hormone DHEA, so long term use of DHEA (greater than four to six months) to support creating a viable pregnancy is not supported and can cause more hormone imbalance and potentially issues in becoming pregnant.

COMMONLY OVERLOOKED: CELIAC DISEASE OR GLUTEN SENSITIVITY

At the beginning of this chapter, you met Kay, a woman diagnosed with unexplained infertility. After discovering that she has celiac disease, Kay was able to address this through diet and supplementation and finally become pregnant.

What is celiac disease, and how does it impact fertility? Celiac disease develops when the body becomes intolerant to gluten in the foods that we eat. Gluten is used to give structure to many types of baked and processed foods, but for some, it can wreak havoc on the digestive system. For these individuals, gluten can cause inflammation in the gut and decrease nutrient absorption. Basically, over time you can become deficient in certain nutrients, and this can be life threatening for some; for others, it can be a slow descent into less than optimal health and less than optimal fertility.

Joseph and his wife came to see me due to his low sperm count. They had been trying for two years before the doctor suggested he get tested. He was a fit, healthy thirty–year-old, and no one suspected there would be any issues.

When Joseph and his wife saw me, they were in a state of shock. They couldn't understand how he would have low sperm count and low motility. The doctors said IVF was their only option, but the count was so low and the quality of the sperm so poor that they may need to seek out a donor.

I took Joseph through an evaluation, and he didn't have any symptoms that stood out, except fatigue. The fatigue was always there but especially after he ate. He had no bowel issues or any notable flatulence that he admitted to, which can be typical symptoms of celiac disease. But I wanted to rule out everything to try to figure out why he would have such significant issues with his sperm.

Due to his history, I asked the doctor to look at his thyroid, adrenals and testosterone, including celiac antibodies. The doctor almost didn't do the tests, telling Joseph that there wasn't any way he had celiac disease. Joseph persisted, thankfully, because the celiac antibodies came up high. They did an endoscopy to confirm, and, to the doctor's amazement, Joseph had celiac disease.

Joseph struggled to get rid of gluten completely at first, but as he slowly removed the gluten, he slowly noticed the fatigue lifting. Feeling better helped give Joseph the motivation to give up gluten completely, and soon his energy levels were great. He said, "I didn't realize how tired I was and how bad I felt until I started to get rid of the gluten and started to really feel better. It is a phenomenal change."

Typical symptoms of gluten intolerance, celiac disease, or gluten sensitivity are as follows:

- Bloating or cramping after ingesting foods containing gluten
- IBS symptoms, constipation, and diarrhea
- Constant low energy
- Deficiency of nutrients noted via blood tests
- Foul-smelling stools

Some people do not have any outward symptoms of celiac disease but may experience the following:

- Fertility issues
- Recurrent miscarriage
- Unexplained anemia or low iron or ferritin levels
- Chronic health issues that don't seem to resolve with proper treatment, such as inflammation of the prostate or urinary tract issues

If blood tests show low iron or ferritin (iron stores) and elevated liver enzymes, this is often a telltale sign that a person may be reacting to gluten.

Blood tests for specific celiac antibodies are as follows:

- Anti-gliadin antibodies
- Anti-transglutaminase antibodies*

- Anti-endomysium antibodies

  * considered to be the most sensitive test

The only way for a definitive diagnosis of celiac disease is to have an endoscopy. This is where a physician puts an instrument down your throat and has a look at your small intestine. A biopsy, or piece of tissue, is taken and examined to see if certain structures called villi are damaged. Sometimes the endoscopy is avoided if the blood tests are positive, and gluten is simply removed from the diet.

NO CELIAC DISEASE: DO I STILL REMOVE GLUTEN?

Sensitivity to gluten can also be an issue if you present with any of these symptoms or test results:

- Bloating or cramping after ingesting foods containing gluten
- IBS symptoms, constipation, and diarrhea
- Deficiency of nutrients
- Foul-smelling stools
- Excessive flatulence
- Unexplained anemia or low iron or ferritin levels
- Elevated liver enzymes
- Elevated thyroid antibodies
- Thyroid or adrenal issues with no clear cause

If these symptoms continue to occur despite taking probiotics, then I suggest removing gluten, even though tests may not be positive for celiac antibodies. Most people notice their symptoms lessening as a result.

Most times though removing gluten is not enough. Working to restore gut health is very important. Studies have revealed that the damage in the gut of those with celiac disease who remove gluten completely still remains but that is likely due to either a poor eating plan without gluten or not working to restore healthy gut function and repair damage in the gut after removing gluten. I usually recommend an herbal protocol with herbs that contain cooling, anti-inflammatory mucilage herbs for restoration of the gut as well as high quality and potency probiotics.

LACTOSE INTOLERANCE

Since we are on the topic of digestion, the issue of lactose intolerance should be assessed and addressed as a possible cause of digestive issues that can impact fertility. Most times, patients are aware of their intolerance to lactose before presenting themselves at the clinic and have already removed the dairy products that irritate them. However, some who enjoy the taste of dairy products, even though they may cause irritation, continue to have these products without realizing how it could impact digestion and nutrient absorption.

If it is common for you to experience loose stools or excessive foul-smelling bowel movements or flatulence, headaches, abdominal bloating, and discomfort with milk products, then avoiding dairy (especially cow's milk) may be a good idea for you to improve your gut health.

Remember, any time you improve your gut health, you will also be improving your fertility. If your gut health is compromised due to inflammation or damage from foods that don't agree with you, it will be more difficult for your body to break down the foods you are eating and absorb nutrients optimally. You need an abundance of nutrients available to the cells in the body (which includes the egg cell and sperm cells) to optimize your health and fertility.

MALE FERTILITY IGNORED

Another common area that is ignored frequently by medical practitioners is male fertility. Patients have come to the clinic and reported their doctors have said the semen analysis was perfectly fine, only to find out after reviewing it that there are issues with quantity or quality that were ignored.

When a woman goes through IVF and the egg fertilizes, it is common for all the responsibility for whether that embryo continues to develop or whether it implants to be placed squarely on the shoulders of the female. Thankfully, through more research, it has been shown that this old opinion is not true. Both the sperm and the egg contribute to the development of the embryo, its implantation, and its continued development once it implants.

A study from Huntsman Cancer Institute (HCI) at the University of Utah reveals that the father's sperm delivers much more complex genetic material than previously thought. It used to be considered that the sperm's only responsibility was to fertilize the egg. However, new research shows that the sperm contributes just as much to the development of the embryo as the egg does. Therefore, if the embryos aren't developing or attaching, male fertility should be looked at and, even if the semen analysis is normal, overall cellular health for the male should be optimized. DNA fragmentation of the sperm is often an issue that is not tested but potentially contributing to poor outcomes with IVF. DNA fragmentation can be an issue even if the semen analysis is normal.

In some mainstream medical circles, it is believed that not much can be done about male fertility issues, and this is possibly the reason it is often ignored. There is no magic pill to fix it. But thankfully because the sperm are just cells like every other cell in the body, there are many ways that it can be addressed and improvement seen, not just in quantity but in quality, as well.

A word about semen analysis:

Make sure the semen analysis is done at an IVF clinic and the analysis includes count and a breakdown of motility and morphology. Unfortunately even IVF clinics don't often perform detailed semen analysis but there is a better chance that an IVF clinic will look at more parameters than a general lab.

Have a wash or prep of the sperm done to see if the count significantly drops. In my patients, a dropping count after the wash has correlated with poorer quality sperm and difficulty getting pregnant naturally or with IVF.

If a semen analysis turns out to be normal and fertility issues persist, a DNA fragmentation test may be necessary to look at the DNA of the sperm. If after testing DNA fragmentation, everything seems to be fine with the sperm but a viable conception is not happening, it is still vitally important that the male follow the Five-Step Fertility Solution™ as well. Semen analysis and blood tests are limited. A doctor or scientist can't determine whether a normal looking sperm has chromosomal abnormalities just from looking at it, just like they can't determine if a normal looking egg has chromosomal abnormalities just by looking at it.

CHROMOSOMAL ISSUES ARE A SIGNIFICANT

A small-scale study published in the journal *Biology of Reproduction* as well as a review cited in the *Cytogenic and Genome Research* journal concluded that sperm with motility issues were at increased risk of having chromosomal abnormalities. It is possible that if this type of sperm fertilizes an egg, the embryo would not develop as well or may end up in miscarriage.

Motility issues can also be related to a genetic variation. University of North Carolina research discovered a variation of the enzyme Choline Dehydrogenase (CHDH) in some men can be associated with motility issues. These men need additional choline through a supplementation program and diet for motility to improve. This is important news. Oftentimes if there is a motility issue with the sperm a procedure called ICSI will be performed which adds potentially unnecessary expense to the IVF procedure when simply diet and supplementation could improve the sperm's ability to travel to the egg. In men without this gene variation, the Five Step Fertility Solution will work extremely well due to an increase in selenium, zinc, vitamin E and other nutrients as well as a decrease in inflammatory processed foods and drinks. With simple straightforward changes we see the motility improve.

A WORD ABOUT ICSI

ICSI, or intracytoplasmic sperm injection, is a technique where a scientist chooses one sperm, and this sperm is then injected into the egg to create a fertilized egg that could develop into an embryo.

This technique is often used to bypass severe issues with the sperm in the hope that it will increase the chances for a fertilization of the egg and subsequently a viable conception. This technique, as well as washing the sperm, has been touted as how IVF can overcome male factor fertility issues. ICSI is also used with more mature females because it is assumed that their eggs are older and may be harder to fertilize. Subsequently, ICIS has been used in increasing numbers over the years.

It's important to keep in mind some things when utilizing ICIS:

- ICIS does appear to increase fertilization rates but does not appear to increase take-home baby rates. Despite its increase in use and increased costs associated with it, research has revealed that ICSI does not appear to be helpful in creating a viable pregnancy no matter what the diagnosis.
- ICIS completely removes any natural selection. If a sperm is not able to fertilize an egg on its own, perhaps it is the health of the sperm that is preventing it from fertilizing the egg and contributing to the development of a healthy embryo. Oftentimes, only the egg is considered to be the problem, and the possibility that the health of the sperm could be the issue is ignored. The truth is, unless they come up with better testing for the egg and the sperm, it is impossible to know.

Therefore, both partners working toward optimizing their fertility appears to make sense.

I find that many couples aren't aware that they have a choice of whether they can use ICIS or not. Some have no idea why ICIS is being used in the first place.

Some couples who have had four or more eggs available to be fertilized have used ICIS on half of the eggs, and the other half were fertilized normally. This is a good compromise for some couples if the physician for some reason is pushing the use of ICSI despite what the research has revealed.

The main point to understand from this section is that the responsibility for creating a baby is not just on the female. It is clear now through research that the sperm's job is not finished after fertilization. The sperm must be healthy enough to contribute to the development of a viable embryo. If an embryo is developing poorly before or after implantation because of an issue with the egg or the sperm, this will likely affect the embryo's survival in the uterus. Failure to implant is not always an issue with the woman's uterus; it can be an issue with the health of the embryo.

RECOMMENDED BLOOD TESTS FOR UNEXPLAINED OR UNRESOLVED FERTILITY ISSUES

Most physicians will do the basic blood tests on both the male and female to rule out sexually transmitted disease, full blood screen, liver function tests, and so on. These tests are very thorough and comprehensive.

The following are the tests that are helpful to further assess male and female fertility.

For her:
On day two to three of the period

E2 or estradiol
FSH (Follicle Stimulating Hormone)
LH (Luteinizing Hormone)
Prolactin
TSH (Thyroid Stimulating Hormone)
FT3
FT4
Reverse T3
Thyroid antibodies

Seven days after ovulation
Progesterone
Estradiol
FSH
LH
Homocysteine (fasting)
Celiac antibodies
AM cortisol (taken in the morning preferably before 9 a.m.)
Vitamin D
DHEA
Cholesterol/triglycerides (fasting)
Urinary iodine (optional but helpful)
Saliva: Cortisol and DHEA and if several IVF cycles, consider looking at salivary estrogens (E1, E2, E3), progesterone, testosterone, DHEA, cortisol through the cycle. Can be ordered by a clinician or without a script in the USA at canaryclub.org

For him (no particular day but try to avoid if sick or on antibiotics)
Free testosterone
Total testosterone
LH (Luteinizing Hormone)
FSH (Follicle Stimulating Hormone)

Estradiol (If increased conversion of testosterone to estrogen is suspected)

Homocysteine (fasting)

TSH (Thyroid Stimulating Hormone)

Free T4

Free T3

Reverse T3

Urinary iodine levels (optional but can be helpful)

Iron studies

Celiac antibodies

Cholesterol/triglycerides (fasting)

Saliva: Testosterone, E1, E2, DHEA, cortisol

In addition to the above tests, I would suggest a semen analysis after six months of timed intercourse and no viable pregnancy, one or more miscarriages, or three months after beginning a program to help optimize male fertility. Please ask for count, breakdown of motility, and morphology to be tested.

If no implantation with IVF after one to two transfers, no pregnancy after twelve months of timed intercourse, or more than one miscarriage, I suggest to determine the health of the DNA with a DNA fragmentation test.

Consider joining the membership site for those trying to conceive at tipstogetpregnant.com.

Our Fertility Membership Site Platinum level includes a *free* fertility herbal formula to begin resetting your system. Tipstogetpregnant.com

Tipstogetpregnant.com offers…

Over 10 hours of webinars (videos) and audios to help men and women dealing with fertility issues.

It includes specific information on fertility related topics such as

➤ Polycystic ovaries

All you need to know to optimize your chances to conceive with PCO

> ➢ Endometriosis

Comprehensive guide to how endometriosis may have developed, how you can address it, and what you can do to keep it from coming back

> ➢ Fertility over forty

An eBook dedicated to helping more mature couples conceive (technically appropriate for anyone over thirty-five)

> ➢ Recurrent miscarriages

Stop the losses and create a viable pregnancy

> ➢ Male fertility solutions

Simple, easy-to-follow steps to improve male fertility

> ➢ Updates to the Five-Step Fertility Solution

When new research comes out, you will be the first to receive it.

> ➢ Audio programs such as How to Get Off The Emotional Rollercoaster and Finding Your Life Again When Dealing With Fertility Issues
> ➢ Closed Facebook Group

You can discuss your fertility issues privately and find support from a community.

To Contact Stacey "The Baby Maker"™ for one-on-one consultations, e-mail info@naturalfertility.com.

You can find a list of practitioners who have graduated from Stacey's Fertility Mentoring Program at tipstogetpregnant.com under the Experts tab.

Practitioners who would like to become an expert on helping men and women dealing with fertility issues please see thebabymakernetwork.com

I would just like to take a moment to wish you all the best on your journey. I know it can be difficult, to say the least, and I truly do wish you all the very best and hope that *The Baby Maker's Guide* has given you a framework to create the little life you long for!

Sincerely,
Stacey "The Baby Maker" Roberts PT, MH, Naturopath

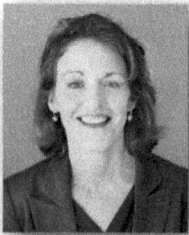

SUMMARY OF HOW I CAN HELP YOU:

SUMMARY OF WHERE you can find additional information:

Men and women dealing with fertility issues or wanting to improve their health to increase their chances of starting a family, please visit the following websites:

Naturalfertility.com (individual consultations)

Tiptogetpregnant.com (membership site and free fertility herbs)

Practitioners:

If you are a practitioner wanting to help couples with fertility issues, go to thebabymakernetwork.com or contact thebaby-maker@naturalfertility.com.

Baby Maker™ Network for Practitioners: An international network of practitioners trained specifically in the Five-Step Fertility Solution. A membership allows a practitioner to learn from over sixty hours of audio and video related to all aspects of fertility: Ten modules covering PCOS, Endometriosis, Male Fertility, Unexplained Fertility, Recurrent Miscarriage, Secondary Fertility, Support During IVF, Fibroids, Tubal Blockages, and more. Contact Stacey "The Baby Maker" at thebabymaker@naturalfertility.com for more information.